Confronting Alzheimer's Disease

Confronting Alzheimer's Disease

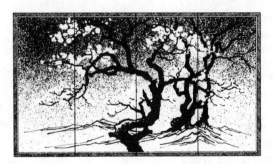

Edited by Anne C. Kalicki, MSc

Published by National Health Publishing
in cooperation with
the American Association of Homes for the Aging

Contents

Contributors

Marion Roach, BS

Marion Roach is the daughter of an Alzheimer's patient and author of *Another Name for Madness* (Boston: Houghton Mifflin, 1985). She lives in New York City.

Burton V. Reifler, MD, MPH

Dr. Burton V. Reifler is Director of the University of Washington's Alzheimer's Research Program in Seattle, Washington.

Nancy N. Dubler, LLB

Nancy N. Dubler is Director of the Division of Legal and Ethical Issues in Health Care at Montefiore Medical Center in the Bronx, New York.

Lissy F. Jarvik, MD, PhD

Dr. Lissy F. Jarvik is Chief of the Section on Neuropsychogeriatrics in the Department of Psychiatry and Behavorial Sciences at UCLA School of Medicine in Los Angeles, California and Chief, Psychogeriatric Unit, West Los Angeles Veterans Administration Medical Center, Brentwood Division.

Jacob Reingold, MS

Jacob Reingold is Executive Vice President of The Hebrew Home for the Aged at Riverdale, New York.

Daniel Sands, PhD

Dr. Daniel Sands is Executive Director of the South Coast Institute for Applied Gerontology in Costa Mesa, California.

Herbert R. Karp, MD

Dr. Herbert R. Karp is Director of Medical Services at Wesley Woods Center and Director of the Division of Geriatric Medicine, Emory University School of Medicine, Atlanta, Georgia.

Charles M. Gaitz, MD

Dr. Charles M. Gaitz is Medical Director of the Geropsychiatry Program of the Houston Geriatric Center and Clinical Professor in the Department of Psychiatry at Baylor College of Medicine in Houston, Texas.

Nancy L. Wilson, MA

Nancy L. Wilson, is an instructor in the Geriatric Program of the Department of Medicine at Baylor College of Medicine in Houston, Texas.

Hazel Mummah-Castillo, RN, MA

Hazel Mummah-Castillo was formerly Director of the Alzheimer's Unit of St. John of God Nursing Hospital and Residence and is a consultant in gerontologic health care in Walnut, California.

Cynthia J. Wallace, RN, MA

Cynthia J. Wallace is Administrator of Morningside House Nursing Home, Inc. in the Bronx, New York.

Audrey S. Weiner, MPH

Audrey S. Weiner is Assistant Administrator of The Hebrew Home for the Aged at Riverdale, New York.

Steven H. Zarit, PhD

Dr. Steven H. Zarit is Professor of Human Development in the Department of Individual and Family Studies and Assistant Director of the Gerontology Center in the College of Human

Development at Pennsylvania State University in University Park, Pennsylvania.

Barbara J. Esposito, RN, BS, MS

Barbara J. Esposito is a psychiatric clinical nurse specialist and was formerly coordinator of dementia programs at the Jewish Home for the Elderly of Fairfield County in Fairfield, Connecticut.

Charles Silverman, AIA

Charles Silverman, is Director of Institutional Programs for the architectural engineering firm of Daniel Mann Johnson Mendenhall in San Francisco, California.

Lorraine G. Hiatt, PhD

Dr. Lorraine G. Hiatt is a consulting environmental psychologist and gerontologist, based in New York City.

Joan Scharf, MSW, ACSW

Joan Scharf is Director of the Adult Day Care Center of the Menorah Park Center for the Aging in Beachwood, Ohio.

Gloria Levine, RN, BSN

Gloria Levine is Director of the Adult Day Care Program for Memory Impaired of the Menorah Park Center for the Aging in Beachwood, Ohio.

Preface

Confronting Alzheimer's Disease stems from an intensive seminar by that name presented at the 24th Annual Meeting of the American Association of Homes for the Aging (AAHA). The seminar brought together a unique combination of national experts: authorities on legal, medical, social, and design issues relating to Alzheimer's disease and other forms of senile dementia, and an impressive array of the pioneering practitioners who have developed special care units in homes for the aging, most especially for treatment of Alzheimer's patients and those with related disorders.

The American Association of Homes for the Aging wishes to express gratitude for the support from The Hebrew Home for the Aged at Riverdale, Bronx, New York, and The Brookdale Foundation, that enabled us to prepare this book.

Confronting Alzheimer's Disease is not a transcript of the proceedings. Rather some of the intensive seminar speakers provided written versions of their remarks; others agreed to have the transcripts of their talks edited into straightforward and concise chapter form.

It is AAHA's hope that the book will provide a thoroughly researched but not overly technical presentation of issues and practical information that will be as useful to any family concerned about Alzheimer's disease and related disorders as it is to administrators and caregivers in the field of health care and services for the aging.

Marion Roach's stirring personal account of the agonies and rewards of dealing with her mother's dementia is a fitting introduction to a volume dealing with efforts to meet the needs she has so eloquently exposed.

Dr. Burton V. Reifler offers hope for improved treatment for Alzheimer's disease in the future in his description of the short history of knowledge about Alzheimer's in Chapter 1. In Chapter 2, Nancy N. Dubler gives a remarkably clear presentation of the murky legal and ethical dilemmas facing Alzheimer's patients and their families.

In Chapter 3, Dr. Lissy F. Jarvik untangles the complexities of diagnosing Alzheimer's and differentiating it from other dementias and other disorders with similar symptoms. Any family confused by a relative's uncertain medical diagnosis should find Dr. Jarvik's essay especially pertinent and helpful.

Patient care is the focus of Chapter 4. Jacob Reingold describes the dramatic changes in the population of nursing homes as people live longer, enter facilities at a later age, and, though frail, are often more mentally than physically indisposed. Dr. Daniel Sands follows with a discussion of the philosophy of care that emphasizes personal dignity and continued growth and learning for each individual. Dr. Herbert R. Karp notes the importance of health care teams who work with family as well as patient, and Dr. Charles M. Gaitz and Nancy L. Wilson elaborate on the organization of comprehensive and interdisciplinary services for patient care.

Chapter 5 gets to the heart of the practical problem solving that developing a special unit for Alzheimer's patients entails. Administrators and families alike should be helped by the experiences and successes described by Hazel Mummah-Castillo of St. John of God Nursing Hospital and Residence of Los Angeles, and by Cynthia J. Wallace of Morningside House Nursing Home in New York City. Audrey S. Weiner follows with a summary of a nationwide survey of special care units that is a gold mine of information about the goals, admission criteria, environmental modifications, staffing, family involvement, programs, and activities in such units.

Care for the caregiver is the focus of Chapter 6. Dr. Steven H. Zarit provides an excellent description of the burden that family members, especially spouses, undertake when caring for Alzheimer's patients, and Barbara J. Esposito offers case examples of the special difficulties of the offspring of Alzheimer's patients, often marked by unresolved relationship issues left over from childhood.

Environmental modifications that make the patient's world more comprehensible as mental faculties deteriorate are described in Chapter 7 where Charles Silverman discusses passive design and an open space concept, and Dr. Lorraine G. Hiatt demonstrates a step-by-step approach to conceiving and designing an appropriate environment for the person afflicted with Alzheimer's disease. It is clear that overmedication and physical restraints can both become unnecessary when sufficiently skilled staff work with a practical and inexpensive design system that permits wandering, facilitates patient monitoring, and promotes patient safety.

Joan Scharf and Gloria Levine of Menorah Park Center for the Aging in Beachwood, Ohio, describe the advantages and practical aspects of providing adult day care at a facility otherwise devoted to long-term care of its residents. Adult day care offers respite for family caregivers of local community residents.

Looking to the future, Jacob Reingold's concluding chapter pinpoints the need for more—and more specialized—facilities for Alzheimer's patients and focuses on the critical importance of staff education within each facility.

The goal of every contributor and of this volume as a whole is to help develop an educated public and a professional core of specialists in the care of America's two and one-half million citizens suffering from Alzheimer's and related disorders.

Introduction

Another Name for Madness

Marion Roach

Seven years ago, my doctor told me that he thought my mother was becoming senile. I thought she was going mad. We were both wrong. My mother is one of more than two million Alzheimer's disease patients in this country. She is having her dignity wrenched from her. I often say that she is losing her mind in handfuls.

What I called madness began as forgetfulness: her keys, the phone number at the house we shared. What I called madness developed into severe depression and vast memory lapses, confusion, and loss of her previous articulate nature. She groped for words and familiar phrases like a partially blind person reeling in the half light of dusk, but to myself I called it madness.

A lot of people both within and outside of the Alzheimer's field, both friends and experts, criticized me for the title of my book: *Another Name for Madness* (New York: Houghton Mifflin, 1985). I fought the title initially, did not like the name, the word madness. It made me uncomfortable, but no longer.

How old was I when I first heard the phrase, "ignorance is bliss"? I have no idea, but I know I was very young. We apply that phrase to romance, and romance is love. But it is not blissful to be ignorant when someone you love is dying of something you do not understand. It is not blissful to be ignorant when, with understanding, you can help someone you love. How old were we when we first learned the sentence, "the truth hurts"? I thought I knew the true impact of both of those lopsided truisms before I truly understood their liabilities.

What in ignorance and pain I first called madness has a proper name, and now I know what it is: Alzheimer's disease. The truth does hurt. It hurts more each time we caregivers feel it. As when I first went away from home to sleep overnight at a friend's house, or first went off to camp, or first went to college at 18, I have had to learn again about separation.

Alzheimer's is a disease of separation. Two years ago, my friend and my mother's doctor, Dr. Barry Reisberg, said something to me that made more sense than any clinical scale or newspaper article or researcher's report. I was pleading for advice. The doctor said, "When the communication stops, the grief begins." That's what separation is all about.

I remember saying to my mother, "Hi Mom, how are you?" and she said, "What day is it?" and I said, "Oh Mom, I have the flu," and she said, "What day is it? What time is it?"

She could not understand, and I could not understand what she was going through. I wrote in my book, almost a year before Dr. Reisberg spoke to me about grief and communication, that grief is a mute sense of panic. I was terribly misunderstanding at first. I did not understand that I was beginning to separate from someone I loved very much.

Alzheimer's is a disease during which those who care most get less and less advice from the person who knows better than anyone how awful this disease is—the one undergoing it.

The diseased persons become less and less able to reveal their panic as they get more sick. And we, the family, the nurse, the caretaker, the husband, the daughter, the wife can be left so very alone and ignorant unless we find help.

In the early stages of my mother's illness, I called her behavior "madness." I was ignorant, but I was also hiding from what I did not want to know. My mother, this wonderful woman who raised me, had not led an extraordinary life, and somehow I did not expect her to have anything extraordinary happen to her. Let me tell you about the mother I knew.

My mother's name is Allene. She is a descendant of Ethan Allen, the Revolutionary War hero; since everyone on her paternal side had Allen in his or her name, her parents made up the name Allene for her.

She was an independent, willful, and witty child. Just as she could toss out phrases and be clever, she could toss on clothes and be beautiful.

She grew up as an only child. Her mother sewed prom dresses for her so that this sleek 17-year-old would never have to be confronted at a dance by another girl in the same dress. My mother would pluck the satin rosettes off her shoulder, put them in her bag when she went out because she didn't like flounces, pin them back on to her shoulders before she got home, and sneak past her mother.

She went on to graduate from the University of Colorado with a degree in journalism and to become a newspaper reporter, a wife, a girl scout leader, a visiting nurse volunteer, and a truly remarkable mother.

We used to sail together. She got me a boat when I was 13, and I raced and sailed and mooned around the same dock that she had sailed from as a girl. One night a week in the summers we would race together, hunched down eating tunafish sandwiches, delicately adjusting the sheets and the sails.

We would race my bluejay, and she would tell me about the nimblet that she had raced at my age. Her boat was lost in a hurricane, so "Always tie it this way," she would say as she demonstrated, "the way I did when I was your age." But she was my age! She was with me, racing with me, and we were both in blue jackets and both wet. When the wind would pick up and the boat would heel way over, we balanced together on the rail with our toes tucked onto the centerboard trunk; we leaned way out over the water, daring the water to curl up and get us.

She would be in front, the first to get wet. I would steady the tiller, inching us closer to the wind, a delicate balance of love and speed. And we laughed and whooped when the wind backed around and tossed us into the cabin. We got a lot of bruises on our matching kneecaps, and we were pals.

I used to play basketball in high school. I had bad knees and wore a combination of arrangements on my knee, a dead giveaway to the opposition. Once a girl ran up to me in a game and kicked me squarely on the right kneecap. I was in agony. My mother flew off the bleachers. I remember the remarkable echo in the gym, the screaming, and the fact that she never seemed to touch a step. She pulled at the referee, shouted at the girl, and shouted at me to defend myself. This was my mother! Later when the girl was making a lap at the opposite end, I applied some pressure with my sneaker to the girl's ankle. When they carried the wailing and shrieking 15-year-old off the court, my mother looked out under her arched eyebrows and gave me just the hint of a smile.

Her kid—she was competitive as hell. My mother went on to get a master's degree in education and to become a teacher at a bilingual preschool on the lower east side of Manhattan. It was a few years after that that she became slightly confused. In time she was reduced to a clerical position in her school, and eventually she had to leave her job.

In the progression of her disease, she became frightened, angry, paranoid, hostile, and incompetent. She became completely dependent on the aid of others. She could not be left alone. She became repetitive, confused, and agitated. She stopped reading. Now she can no longer form complete sentences. She speaks rapid gibberish. She has no memory, and has to be bathed, fed, and dressed. She lives in a nursing home where total care is provided.

My mother is 57 years old. She seems terribly young to be so terribly ill.

There are no truths to be learned without a challenge to one's courage. I believe that every truth, every success comes after pushing one's courage another distance. In the course of this disease, I have had to learn to push courage into the unknown again and again, despite the panic, the loneliness, and the feeling of total despair.

Right from the start, the Alzheimer's patient and the family must accept the truth of this disease and accept the care available. We learn to do things to prolong the independence of the Alzheimer's patient, to prolong dignity, to prolong the remaining shreds of intellect. We learn to label the drawers on the cabinets, so that the person can dress alone as long as she or he can read.

The word patient has to describe the caregiver. We learn to be patient. We learn to aid as long as we can, until we finally have to do the tasks ourselves. We learn that there is a razor-edged fineness between teaching helplessness and prolonging ability.

We learn a great deal. Five years ago, when my mother was first diagnosed, I looked in a dictionary and found no listing. Then I looked under senile, and the dictionary definition said, "having the characteristics of old age." At the time of the diagnosis, my mother had a cross-court backhand in tennis that would terrify you. She could bowl; she was beautiful; she had an immaculately intelligent look about her.

Next I looked in the encyclopedia, and there was no listing. I finally found in a library an outdated text on neurology that had just half a paragraph.

When my doctor told us of the diagnosis, he began by saying, "Your mother is not going to die." We thought his words were being offered in comfort, in reassurance. Our father had died, and we did not want our mother to suffer, too. We have since learned that the doctor was preparing us with these words for something for which there is no quick end in sight.

Several months after the diagnosis, I decided to write a piece for the *New York Times Magazine.* I was very frightened, but I felt that I could do this. It took me six months to write. Within the first two days after the piece appeared in January of 1983, I received 500 letters. I received over 1,000 phone calls in the five days following publication, and I am still getting letters from it.

It occurred to me that this was a subject on which people wanted to know something. Over 90 percent of the letters were from people with experiences similar to mine. I found it stunning that there was so little known, and yet so many people were being hurt.

I was invited to speak to The Hebrew Home for the Aged at Riverdale shortly after the publication of my magazine piece. I was very bitter at the time, very unhappy, and extremely uncomfortable to be speaking in a nursing home. I was terribly frightened.

I did not want to think that my mother would ever end up in a nursing home; I really thought that that's where people got dumped. I ended up speaking about the economics of the problem, and how it bankrupted my family.

I decided to write a book. It came out in August 1985. I did a nationwide book tour and met hundreds of people; everyone knew someone who had this illness or someone who cared for someone who did. I am still stunned at the numbers.

Things have changed since I first wrote about this. New York City has had its third annual mayoral conference on this subject. November is Alzheimer's Month. That's wonderful. There is a national Alzheimer's Disease and Related Disorders Association. We have research. We've gone to Congress; we're a powerful political force.

One by one we learn and, one step at a time, we do what we can. A year ago, no one could have told me that my mother would be in a nursing home. I fought it. My mother was living in an apartment which my sister and I bought for her with 24-hour-a-day, 7-day-a-week care, at a cost of $4,000 a month. My sister and I had exhausted my father's life savings and my mother's life savings. We were using our salaries to support her, and we were desperate.

I was relentless in my desire to keep my mother out of a home, until I learned a new definition of freedom: the definition of life itself is freedom. By making the decisions every step of the way for my mother, the Alzheimer's patient, I was taking over her freedom and reducing her to a noncontributing person.

I had to reevaluate my feelings about freedom. Before my mother went into the nursing home, she had no freedom and no privacy. She was aided in every aspect of her day, always watched, never alone.

Jacob Reingold, who has become a very good friend and who directs at The Hebrew Home for the Aged at Riverdale, happened to call me right about this time. He said "Why don't you come up here? You didn't look very happy that time you made that speech here; why don't you come up and let me show you around my facility?"

We had lunch and talked; I spent four hours with him. We sat in his office, and I started to cry. He took my hands and said, "You know, you've done a very good job, your sister and you, you've protected your mother. She's safe. But when the nurse gets finished cleaning, dressing, and feeding your mother, do you really think she has any time to talk to her?"

He said, "Come on, let's try a nursing home and see what happens. Let us in the field of caring see what we can do."

What I learned was that my mother had the right to a less restricted environment. You could not have told me two years ago that that would be a nursing home, but it is.

In the apartment, she was being heavily sedated; she had no stimulation. The people we paid were just keeping her fed and dressed; they were not paid to keep her stimulated.

I put my mother in the nursing home. The anticipation of the experience was as far from the reality as is, I hope, anticipating one's own death.

I was very unhappy. What I feared most was leaving her there—leaving her there to live or to die. I brought forms that released her brain to autopsy when she dies.

When my mother went into the home, she was not speaking, she could not recognize me, she barely walked. She seemed dead. On her second day in that nursing home, my mother initiated a conversation for the first time in six months. She recognized me, and she still recognizes me, a year and two months later.

She is happy, cared for, stimulated, safe, and clean. She speaks to me; I would not trade that for anything in the world. Her sedation is half what it was. Professionals work with her every day to keep her stimulated with art therapy, dance therapy, music therapy, and current events. Mental stimulation is her right as a human being; she is fulfilled.

I am grateful beyond words for the help that my mother has received. My hope is that everyone with Alzheimer's can be enabled to have that kind of care, that quality of care.

Chapter 1

A Strange, Eventful History

Burton V. Reifler

Almost 400 years ago, William Shakespeare may have been describing an individual with Alzheimer's disease when he gave Jacques, the acerbic philosopher in *As You Like It*, his famous lines about the seven ages of man. Jacques ends with the aging man:

> Last scene of all,
> That ends this strange eventful history,
> Is second childishness, and mere oblivion,
> Sans teeth, sans eyes, sans taste, sans everything.

We know today that what Shakespeare described is not a normal part of an individual's life; it is a disease—Alzheimer's disease. Even a few decades ago, we did not know that Shakespeare's "second childishness" was a diagnosable illness.

What has the course of our knowledge on Alzheimer's been over the last several decades? In the 1950s, we first began to see descriptions of the number of patients with dementia. What studies there were came from the United Kingdom. Prior to that, there had been very little research on the epidemiology of mental illness in old age. Research began by counting the numbers of patients with the different mental disorders of old age—what was then called senility, depression, alcoholism, and so on.

Two major developments occurred in the 1960s that allowed us to abandon the concept of senility, which suggested a normal loss of memory as people age, in favor of a disease concept of memory loss in old age. The first development was the discovery that pathologic changes in the brains of individuals with progressive loss of memory were the same for people over 60 as for those under 60.

When I was a medical student, I had been taught that Alzheimer's disease applied to people under the age of 60. If you were over 65, you had senile dementia. If you were between 60 and 65, there was no good term that applied to you.

The second development in the 1960s was the realization that Alzheimer's disease was due neither to poor blood supply nor to hardening of the arteries, arteriosclerosis. Blood flow studies, done primarily in Scandinavia, showed that individuals with this gradual, progressive loss of memory that we would now call Alzheimer's disease, had normal circulation to the brain. And when the circulation to the brain became abnormal, the abnormality was a result of the disease rather than a cause of the disease.

These findings made us realize that most old people are doing just fine, but that a very significant minority undergo progressive loss of mental function.

Two other major developments occurred in the 1970s. The most exciting was the detection of specific neurochemical abnormalities in the brains of Alzheimer's patients. They gave us hope that perhaps we were dealing with a situation analogous to Parkinson's disease, where there was a deficiency of a specific chemical—dopamine—and medication that replaced dopamine had been found to provide much improved treatment to patients. But we have not been able to have that success with Alzheimer's. We have not figured out how to correct those neurochemical abnormalities.

The second major development in the 1970s was a focus on diagnosis and therapy: namely, making an accurate diagnosis of Alzheimer's disease and conducting a thorough evaluation of the patient to look for other coexisting illnesses that might be worsening the Alzheimer's.

One fundamental abnormality seems to be a deficiency of acetylcholine. The places where acetylcholine should attach in order to get its message from the sending cell to the receiving cell seem to be intact. This may hold great hope for the future. My prediction is that within the next decade we will see greatly improved treatment for Alzheimer's disease based on correcting these chemical abnormalities.

I do not expect a cure for Alzheimer's: it would take unprecedented good fortune to discover such a cure. Very few chronic diseases have been proven curable.

In the 1980s, there has been an enormous increase in the research base and also in clinical programs on Alzheimer's disease. Our Alzheimer's clinic at the University of Washington, which I established in 1978, was the first clinic of its kind on the west coast. Now virtually every large city with a medical school has some sort of Alzheimer's clinic.

Today, there is a national organization of family support groups, the Alzheimer's Disease and Related Disorders Association (ADRDA), and there are research centers specifically for Alzheimer's disease, funded by both the National Institute of Mental Health and the National Institute on Aging.

In a nutshell, the major developments are:

- accurate diagnosis
- enormously expanded research activities
- the detection of specific chemical abnormalities
- improvements in the recognition of coexisting illnesses that can be treated to good advantage.

Facilities can deal with Alzheimer's disease in eight ways.

1. *Be accessible to Alzheimer's patients and to their families.* Individuals are often willing to go to great lengths to reach the lofty tower of understanding of this complex disease. Sometimes in our care facilities or hospitals, we place needless barriers between the application process and the individual receiving care. We have to be accessible to the demented elderly.

One move in the right direction may be specialized Alzheimer's units in nursing homes. These units can increase our availability and our receptiveness to Alzheimer's patients.

There was a time when a family caring for an Alzheimer's patient would call a nursing home for help, and when the intake person learned that the diagnosis was Alzheimer's disease, there would be a long pause on the phone and the reply to the family would be, "Well, we will get back to you as soon as we can," or "Well, we do not accept Alzheimer's patients in our nursing home." That is nonsense: if you can show me nursing homes that claim they have no Alzheimer's patients, I will come and personally evaluate every patient in the facilities if they will make a donation of $1,000 to our research fund for every Alzheimer's patient I find.

Sometimes, of course, patients with Alzheimer's disease are admitted to a nursing home under other names such as "chronic brain syndrome," "organic brain syndrome," or "arteriosclerosis."

Whatever you call the problem, the point is to be accessible from the start to Alzheimer's patients and their families.

2. *See Alzheimer's patients as individuals and develop an individual treatment plan.* We each perceive an individual with different preconceived ideas about him or her. One person sees someone who is mentally impaired, unable to do normal, daily activities; another sees someone with a chronic illness who may have some difficulty getting around but with appropriate services can remain in the community and manage daily activities adequately.

The point, of course, is that we cannot rely on our stereotypes. We must find out the details of this individual's situation and establish a treatment plan based on those unique considerations.

Picasso's *Old Guitarist* depicts a man who probably has a spinal deformity. We know nothing about his cognitive function. Is he demented, or is his mental function intact?

We do not know. We have to do an evaluation. He may be perfectly able to play the guitar, or he may have difficulties.

In my judgment, there are effective treatment approaches at every stage of Alzheimer's disease. Ten years ago, I would have given physicians points for making an accurate diagnosis of Alzheimer's, but today that is not enough. Today we have the capacity to establish a treatment plan based on the accurate diagnosis.

In our own setting for example, we investigate a list of categories on every patient we see to consider what recommendations for treatment we can make:

a. Stopping or starting medication. Stopping medication is first on the list. As a physician, I have no hesitation about starting a medication if I think it can help. Patients with Alzheimer's disease may be depressed or paranoid. In those and other situations, medication can be helpful, but I think we have helped more people by taking them off drugs than by starting them on new drugs.

b. Medical treatment for coexisting illnesses. I will get back to this subject shortly.

c. Environmental changes.

d. Counseling for the patient and the family.

e. Additional help.

f. Community programs, such as adult day centers. There is a growing trend within nursing homes to establish what Josh Gortler, director of the Caroline Kline Galland Home in Seattle, has called an in-house day care program, a structured, daily activity program for Alzheimer's patients in the nursing home.

g. Respite for the caregiver.

h. Legal and financial arrangements.

i. Referral to the local chapter of ADRDA, the Alzheimer's Disease and Related Disorders Association.

j. Research participation, which often gives the families, and frequently even the patients, the sense that they are contributing to an eventual cure, not just sitting on the sidelines waiting for something to happen but actively engaging in the struggle to combat Alzheimer's disease. Even if the involvement may not help them directly, they take consolation in the fact that it may help future generations.

Evaluating these criteria for each Alzheimer's patient helps the caregiver develop an individual treatment plan.

3. *Assist the families of Alzheimer's patients.* Alzheimer's families usually want to reach out and try to help the patient, but it is hard for them to know what to do.

Alzheimer's programs in nursing homes should be attentive to the needs of families as well as to the needs of the residents. Sometimes the best help that we can give a family is to suggest what they see as *less* help. If they are coming out two and three times a day to feed the patient every meal, they are exhausting themselves and interfering with daily routines. Sometimes our most helpful suggestion is to set up a specific visiting schedule.

4. *Remove sources of excess disability.* I was recently involved in a research project for which the primary investigator was Eric Larson, my colleague in the Department of Medicine at the University of Washington.

In diagnostic evaluations of 107 patients, almost all of whom had Alzheimer's disease, we found numerous coexisting illnesses. Twenty-nine out of the 107 were also depressed. We have replicated this now in several samples; one-quarter to one-third of all Alzheimer's patients are also depressed.

In another study, we are looking at treatment of depression in Alzheimer's patients. Although we have not completed the analysis of all of our data, our preliminary conclusion is that the depression seen in Alzheimer's patients is eminently treatable. If an Alzheimer's patient is depressed, I recommend that you treat the depression. You can expect to see improvement in the individual's spirit and in daily activities. You are not likely to see great improvement in cognitive function. Expect depression to improve; be pleasantly surprised if cognition improves as well.

We divided our patients into two groups. While one group received tricyclic antidepressant medication and the other received placebos, both groups showed improvement in their depression. In other words, antidepressant medication may not be the only treatment for depressed Alzheimer's patients. There may be a number of approaches that can successfully treat an individual's depression.

Alzheimer's patients are at high risk for undetected illnesses. Imagine a man who has a broken leg, but who also carries a ball and chain. The ball and chain could be labeled "excess disability." Obviously, he has an easily correctable source of excess disability. Remove it, and he will still be left with his primary disability, which is his broken leg. For a patient with Alzheimer's disease, depression, overmedication, hypothyroidism, or any coexisting illness can act like a ball and chain. Help each patient to remove those sources of excess disability.

5. *Create a suitable environment for Alzheimer's patients.* When you have people over to entertain, I somehow doubt that you put a row of chairs along one wall, another row of chairs along the other, and then expect to have a nice lively conversation. But I have seen such a configuration in long-term care facilities. In such a setting, the most exciting element of the daily routine is sitting there in the front hallway and seeing who is going to get a visitor. There is room for improvement, preferably with more logically normal living areas where people can mix and mingle and engage in conversation.

There is a somewhat apocryphal story about happy hour at a nursing home. Once a week, staff would offer residents a choice of wine or beer before dinner. A strange thing happened. Even the very demented men would shave and put on a clean shirt about a half hour before happy hour. Even the very demented women would put on makeup and a fresh dress. Staff would play music at the appropriate time, and when people went to the dining area, there seemed to be more conversation over dinner than usual. Unfortunately, the community got wind of it, thought this was a terrible thing, plying these old people with alcohol, and the happy hour was discontinued.

The point to remember is that even a small investment in improving the environment can have a major impact on the patient's sense of well-being.

6. *Keep the patient's interests first.* We can get bogged down in turf battles: "Whose responsibility is it?" "I should be doing this." "No, I should be doing this."

If we become embroiled in turf issues or staff issues, we need to detach ourselves a bit, imagine the attitude of someone seeing us from a great distance away, from a mountain top or another planet. Then we should put those struggles aside and remind ourselves that the patient's interests come first.

7. *Set as your goal teamwork within the facility.* Think of a rowing crew skimming down the Thames. It takes an enormous amount of practice and an enormous amount of teamwork to keep that shell going in a straight line. Each oar has to be providing just the right contribution.

When you see the task done well, it is not obvious how difficult teamwork is. This is one of the problems we face in long-term care facilities. When all is going well and running smoothly, it is not that obvious to an outside observer how much teamwork is involved. Teamwork is only noticeable when it is absent, when we see one oar clank into another.

Several elements are analogous to each of the oars in the shell. We certainly want the patients to have enough help to be able to do daily activities of living, but we do not want them to have more help than they actually need. We do not want to take away any more independence than necessary.

In terms of the medical evaluation, we want the patients to have all necessary tests, but we do not want to subject them to unnecessary procedures. We certainly want to have enough staff time available, yet we do not want to have so much that it becomes counterproductive. Every aspect of an Alzheimer's patient's care in a nursing home deserves attention, and all have to be kept in balance with one another.

8. *Develop your own clear vision of the future.* One of my patients died last week, a well-known industrialist named William Allen; he was head of the Boeing Corporation for about 20 years. William Allen had a sense of vision. He saw that the way of the future in the aircraft industry was the jet aircraft. He staked the company's future on the

707, which was the father of commercial jet transport.

William Allen died of Alzheimer's disease, but although he could no longer remember them in his final years, his great achievements have an enduring impact on this nation's primacy in the field of aircraft engineering.

My final challenge to all caregivers of Alzheimer's patients is to have your own vision of the future, just as Mr. Allen had such a clear vision.

Follow your intuition, your hunches, and do not be afraid to take a well-calculated risk. Remember Sergeant Preston's law: the scenery only changes for the dog in the lead.

Chapter 2

The Legal and Ethical Dilemma

Nancy N. Dubler

Allocating decision-making authority among health care providers, patients, and families is a difficult matter. It is sufficiently complex when it involves someone who is essentially independent and healthy but has been hospitalized for an acute care intervention; it is even complicated when it involves someone who seeks outpatient care with a primary care provider. Decision-making issues, however, become far more convoluted when they arise in the world of Alzheimer's disease. That world includes patient, provider, institution, family, and the state.

This comment will focus on two themes: first, the rights of Alzheimer's patients and, second, the responsibilities of families. The language of rights is strong language and may sound harsh or even foolish when applied to a patient afflicted with this particular disease. Nonetheless, people do not lose rights because of the onset of disability or because they cannot exercise them. With victims of Alzheimer's disease, the language of rights must be softened by concepts of compassion.

In the same fashion, the responsibilities of families should be evaluated bearing in mind each family's range of emotional, intellectual, and financial resources. When dealing with Alzheimer's patients, their providers, and their families, it is appropriate to assume the best of will and good intentions, until one or another is proved false.

11

Rights of Alzheimer's Patients

- the right to know
- the right to grieve
- the right to be supported
- the right to plan for assets
- the right to consider the range of future health care options
- the right to be permitted to participate in research.

The Right to Know

Many Alzheimer's patients, especially those in the early stages of their disease, are aware of a growing disability. Despite these suspicions, there is too often a conspiracy of silence surrounding the care of the Alzheimer's patient, as it used to surround the care of cancer patients.

Ten years ago, when I first began working in health care, some physicians—and there are still some today—would never use the word cancer with their patients; they would talk about a terrible disease or a tumor or substitute some other euphemism. Early work done with cancer patients indicated that the vast majority of physicians who worked with cancer patients assumed their patients did not know they had cancer; needless to say, the vast majority of the patients did in fact know.

My experience, and that of the caregivers with whom I work, indicates that many patients with early Alzheimer's disease are fully aware that something unexplained is happening. They are frightened, anxious, and disoriented.

In the context of health care, the right to provide informed consent or refusal, i.e., to exercise informed choice, requires a patient to consider not only the diagnosis, the prognosis, and the course and conduct of a disease, but also the possible treatments and the projected risks and benefits of each intervention. This right to choose is no less applicable to Alzheimer's patients than to others. The difference lies in the fact that at some time in the disease process the ability to choose will be destroyed.

Law and ethical principles require that patients be told about their condition.Without that knowledge, patients are disempowered. Without that knowledge, others must decide for them. Without that knowledge, there is no way to ferret out, to document, and to give respect to the individual's personal preferences for care.

The doctrine of informed consent is based on two legal pillars. The first is the common-law concept of self-determination, that right which protects an individual's right to decide regarding "what shall be done with his own body." The second is the right to privacy, a constitutional right that protects a sphere of decision making about health care and the use of one's body. It also protects decisions about care in the future when and if the patient can no longer address the issues.

The doctrine of informed consent serves a number of purposes. It guards individual decision making; it protects against fraud and duress; and it ensures the authenticity and individual appropriateness of decisions about care, even those that seem idiosyncratic.

The doctrine of informed consent assumes for its operation that a person is capable of making decisions. Are Alzheimer's patients capable of so doing? Are they able to decide?

Certainly, common sense dictates—the law does not need to tell us—that a patient in the last stage of Alzheimer's disease, who is incontinent of bladder and bowel, who has curled into a fetal position, who no longer recognizes family, and who responds only to pain, is not capable of making decisions.

But there is a time at the beginning and early stages of the disease when many patients can still focus on issues of importance to them. They are still in touch with what I have called their "sedimented life preferences," that is, with those life values and patterns of existence that they developed as adults and that may have survived the ravages of dementia. Are these patients capable of making decisions? Are they competent? What is required for one to be competent?

Competence is a term with a range of meanings. First, it is a legal presumption: we assume that people are competent to make decisions at a certain age. That age used to be 21. When we began drafting men at 18, it seemed ludicrous to have people die for their country at 18 and not be able to vote. So, Congress amended the Constitution to lower the voting rights age to 18. Most state legislatures followed suit and lowered the general age of competence to 18.

A wonderful example of the forces that affect fluctuating notions of the age of competence harks back to the Middle Ages. As the weight of armor increased, the age of competency increased, because in order to be a knight in the army, i.e., an adult, you had to wear armor and fight for the king. Put simply, there is nothing magic about the term *competence*. It is a societal artifact that reflects how we, as a society, choose to do business and whether we choose to empower people within society or to exclude them from full participation.

In the context of health care decisions, however, competence or the capability to make decisions implies something quite different: namely, the ability to have a set of values and to apply those values to a set of options with some understanding of the consequences.

This is a rather rigorous definition, but in the case of Alzheimer's patients, I propose that the definition can be used to describe "decision-specific competence." In order to be capable, a person need not be equally capable of making all decisions, for all purposes, at all times.

An Alzheimer's patient, for example, may exhibit as the first signs of the disease, an inability to manage the very complex financial calculations at which he or she was previously so adept. Although this person can no longer manage a checkbook or act as an accountant, he or she may still have very strong feelings about health care, about life support systems, and about how the family is to care for him or her in the future. The patient may also have strong opinions regarding the disposition of assets.

An Alzheimer's patient has a right to know, because the Alzheimer's patient may still possess decision-specific competence and may therefore still have the right to make certain sorts of decisions. Preferences regarding terminal care and regarding maintenance of life support systems may survive long after mathematical ability or word-finding capacity have diminished.

The Right to Grieve

With the knowledge that something is wrong and the clear dawning of realization that abilities are diminishing, declining, and sliding away, there is grieving. Alzheimer's patients and their families can grieve together. That grieving enables families to give assurances of the sort of care, support, and love they will provide in the future. They can pledge that they will remain constant in the substance of their love. Patients have the right to grieve and to say goodbye. Family members need to be provided with the same opportunity.

The Right to Be Supported

Patients have the right to be supported by health care staff with the latest, the best, and the most appropriate care that modern medicine can offer. The overuse of chemical constraints, such as tranquilizing medications, are sloppy alternatives to appropriately planned and administered long-term care. It is unfair, and a denial of a patient's right to care, to substitute restraints for adequate staffing and for the sort of intelligent facility design that can permit patient movement without risking injury or elopement. It is a denial of a patient's right to care to use segregation and enforced idleness as a substitute for program and stimulation. Limiting, constricting, and confining care for the convenience of staff violate the patient's right to be cared for and supported.

The Right to Plan for Assets

Alzheimer's is not only a devastating disease for the patient personally and for the family emotionally, it is also a disease that can bring total financial devastation to all. Most patients at some point in the course of their disease must enter a long-term care facility. If there has been early and careful financial planning, payment for long-term care will not impoverish the spouse and dependent children. Trust funds can be established that protect assets transferred from the Alzheimer's victim to the spouse; transfer of funds must occur sufficiently early after the onset of symptoms so that the patient, when necessary, can qualify for Medicaid assistance for long-term care.

Most Alzheimer's patients are part of couples who have worked hard and amassed some small savings, perhaps tens of thousands of dollars over a lifetime. If all assets are in the name of the afflicted party, the other will be left destitute in the community. That need not happen. It can only be prevented, however, if, once the diagnosis is made, knowledgeable and careful legal support is secured.

The Right to Consider the Range of Future Health Care Options

In the last decade, there have been several much-publicized law cases that have explored the issues of withdrawing and withholding care from patients who are no longer able to decide for themselves.

The cases began to emerge in 1976 with the case of Karen Ann Quinlan, a 21-year-old woman who was brought into a hospital in respiratory failure and put on a ventilator. Her parents, who were devout Catholics, after consultation with their parish priest and with church legal experts, petitioned the court to have Karen's father appointed as her guardian for the particular purpose of exercising her right to refuse care. Her father stated that he wished to disconnect the respirator and permit Karen to die.

The New Jersey Supreme Court, in that first and very courageous opinion, stated that Karen's constitutional right to privacy would protect her right to refuse treatment were she capable of so doing. The court reasoned that the fact that someone is no longer capable of exercising a right does not mandate the disappearance of that right. It does mean, however, that the questions to be asked are different. We must ask: Who may exercise that right? On what standard? With what procedural safeguards?

The court, in this early case, answered these questions by declaring that a legally appointed guardian should exercise the right. On what standard? The court stipulated a standard of "substituted judgment," that is, what would this patient want if this patient could tell us? In the case of Karen Quinlan, there is a paragraph where the court says that if Karen were magically alive, the court would have no doubt that she would want the respirator turned off. This is rather a flight of fancy on the court's part, as, needless to say, Karen, who was 21, had probably never considered those issues and had certainly not clearly communicated a position. Nonetheless, the court said the crucial standard is individual preference.

The final question concerned issues of procedural regularity. How could this disconnection come about? The court judged that the proper way was to convene a hospital prognosis committee. Once that committee decided that the prognosis was hopeless, then a guardian could be appointed to exercise Karen's right, based upon what she would wish, and, if appropriate, terminate treatment.

The respirator was discontinued, and Karen Quinlan lived for some ten years thereafter, dying in April 1985. In the intervening years, however, many state courts have confronted similar circumstances involving withdrawing or withholding care from one clearly not capable of individual decision. Most of these state courts have stated that the proper standard for choosing the appropriate health care intervention for one who cannot do so is the doctrine of "substituted judgment": What would this person want if this person could tell us?

Now, however, some ten years after the Quinlan case, we have more specific legal instruments that can be used to avoid some of the moral and legal uncertainties that stem from the attempt to guess what a particular patient would want. In the case of the Alzheimer's patient, one reason to involve the patient early on in the course of the disease is to enable the patient to execute either a *living will* or a *durable power of attorney* for health care decisions. These are documents that permit the patient to state explicitly what he or she would want in the event that, in the future, he or she is unable to participate in decisions about health care. Issues such as the appropriateness of respirators, feeding tubes, gastrotomies, even antibiotics (for recurring urinary tract infections, for example, if one is permanently catheterized) can all be addressed by specific instructions in these advance directives.

The form of "advance directives," the generic term for living wills and durable powers of attorney, varies from state to state. Caregivers and nursing home administrators should check with legal services for the elderly or with their facility's attorney to ascertain what specific requirements are necessary in that jurisdiction.

When long-term care administrators help patients to execute these documents—not as they enter the nursing home, nor as they fill in forms on the first day, but somewhere over those first months—they should elicit from patients, if possible, their preferences for care. Some patients will no longer be able to comment. Some, however, whose major problem is wandering, for example, may still be able to focus on preference. For those too debilitated, the family may be able to provide guidance, or in the best instance, a previously executed advance directive.

There is a growing preference for durable powers of attorney over living wills. These documents empower a specific person to communicate the preferences and to execute the desires of the patient. The durable power of attorney provides an advocate for the patient.

In contrast, a living will is a piece of paper. Pieces of paper get lost. They do not get lost as often in long-term care facilities as they do in acute care hospitals, but anyone who has ever tried to find a chart in a major, urban teaching hospital can comprehend qualms about the effectiveness of a living will. Nonetheless, these are easy to obtain, simple to fill out, and, in most jurisdictions, deserving of respect.

An issue increasingly confronting society in general and nursing homes in particular concerns whether it is appropriate to withdraw or withhold food and fluid from end-stage elderly demented, institutionalized patients.

A case in New Jersey decided in January 1984, *In the Matter of Claire Conroy*, focused attention on this issue. The case involved a woman with end-stage dementia who was unresponsive, fed by a nasogastric tube, unable to recognize relatives, and curled into a fetal position. She followed people with her eyes occasionally and sometimes responded with a sort of purr when someone brushed her hair.

Her nephew, who was her legal guardian, petitioned to have the nasogastric tube removed. The court, as in the Quinlan case, asked who may act, on what standard, and with what protections? The court said that nutrition could be withheld on any of three standards:

1. a *subjective standard*, fulfilled when someone has left specific orders regarding the decision under consideration

2. a *limited objective standard,* if it could be told from the way the patient had behaved and the sort of life the patient had led whether or not the patient would not want life to be maintained in a mechanical fashion; additionally, if the continuation of treatment must involve suffering

3. a *pure objective standard,* if there is no benefit to the patient, if the burdens of existence overwhelm the benefit of continued life, and if it is inhumane to continue suffering.

The court then set up specific procedures in New Jersey. The guardian must refer the case to the state ombudsman who must consider every case of withdrawal as a possible case of abuse; the ombudsman must investigate, subpoena, take evidence, and reach a decision.

I find these standards to be challenging and worrisome. American society has not protected our vulnerable populations well, neither the retarded, nor the institutionalized, nor poor children. I query whether we have the moral maturity or the wisdom to develop rules to permit institutions to take measures to withdraw the very sustenance of life from elderly demented patients.

The Right to be Permitted to Participate in Research

Many Alzheimer's patients might like to participate in research. Such participation might imbue their last days of suffering and loss with some meaning beyond their own pain. Currently, enrolling Alzheimer's patients in research is a difficult and problematic matter, as qualification to be a research subject under federal regulations depends on the patient's voluntary informed consent. Alzheimer's patients in the last stages of the disease cannot provide that consent, but patients in the early stages of the disease can. Using a durable power of attorney, a patient could appoint a representative with authority to permit participation in research. Many Alzheimer's patients could consent to long-range, long-term protocols. Use of these designs would permit patients, when capable, to consent to protocols in the future.

Involving Alzheimer's patients early in the course of their disease in discussions about research can do much to enhance society's ability to gain knowledge that could hypothetically benefit future Alzheimer's patients.

Responsibilities of Families of Alzheimer's Patients

The subject of family responsibility must be raised with gentleness and without negative judgments. The families of Alzheimer's patients are often the most stressed, albeit the most loving and caring, of families. They tend to be unclear about their rights and are therefore insufficiently able to fulfill some of their responsibilities.

1. Families have the responsibility to confront the disease with the patient and to participate in grieving.

2. Families have the responsibility to be honest with themselves and with the patient.

3. Families have the responsibility to be courageous, although it is probably up to the caregivers to make this responsibility a possibility.

4. Families have the responsibility to recognize self-interest as valid, to recognize that family members have the right to continue their lives and have the obligation to themselves to do so.

5. Families have the responsibility to plan for a viable continuation of their lives in the community beyond the time when the illness of the Alzheimer's victim will have left them alone.

These rights and responsibilities that I have outlined are very broad. They can only occur when caregivers help people to understand the issues that they face as patient and caregiver. The support of professional caregivers makes discussions of rights and responsibilities possible.

Chapter 3

How Do We Recognize
This Enemy?

Lissy F. Jarvik

What do we know about Alzheimer's disease, the enemy that reduces its victims to mere shadows of their former selves? Do we know where this enemy originates? Do we carry it inside us? Does it attack us from without? Do we know where it hides? Do we know its allies?

We do not know the causes of Alzheimer's disease; most likely, the causes are manifold. We do not know any cures. In some instances, we do not even know how to recognize it. Yet to conquer your enemy you must know your enemy. The purpose of this chapter is to summarize how well we are doing in learning to recognize and diagnose Alzheimer's disease.

Diagnostic Criteria for Alzheimer's Disease

Before we can diagnose Alzheimer's disease, one of the many forms of dementia, we have to make the diagnosis of dementia. The official guidelines of the American Psychiatric Association (1980), as presented in the *Diagnostic and Statistical Manual, Third Edition*

*This work is supported in part by National Institute of Mental Health Research Grant MH36205 and by the Veterans Administration. The author gratefully acknowledges the assistance of Cynthia Pearson, Ph.D., in the preparation of this manuscript. The opinions expressed are those of the author and not necessarily those of the Veterans Administration.

21

(DSM-III), include the key symptoms in four criteria.

The *first criterion* is a loss of intellectual ability of sufficient severity to interfere with social or occupational functioning. It is clear, however, that Alzheimer's disease starts long before the impairment is sufficiently severe to interfere with functioning. Accordingly, we must acknowledge from the outset that our criteria are flawed.

The *second criterion* is memory impairment; however, it is important to remember that not all impairment of memory signals dementia. Not only is a good deal of forgetting within the normal range, but there are many causes of memory impairment other than dementia.

The *third criterion* can be met by any one of the following four symptoms:

- impairment of abstract thinking: as when a person thinks that a statement like "A stitch in time saves nine" pertains only to mending;

- impaired judgment: as when a person withdraws savings from an account on the day before quarterly interest would be credited;

- cortical dysfunction: as when a person exhibits difficulty with calculations, language, and orientation in space;

- personality change: as when a person who is usually trusting becomes very suspicious.

The *fourth criterion* requires that the patient's state of consciousness not be clouded, so that the patient is alert and aware of the surroundings. This criterion is especially important because if consciousness is clouded, then the diagnosis is delirium rather than dementia.

A Work Group on the Diagnosis of Alzheimer's Disease sponsored by the National Institute of Neurological and Communicative Disorders and Stroke (NINCDS) and the Alzheimer's Disease and Related Disorders Association (ADRDA) under the auspices of the U.S. Department of Health and Human Services Task Force on Alzheimer's Disease further refined clinical criteria for the diagnosis of probable, possible, and definite Alzheimer's disease (McKhann et al. 1984).

Criteria for *probable* Alzheimer's disease include dementia cs tablished by clinical examination, with documented mental status, and neuropsychological test confirmation; deficits in two or more areas of cognition; progressive worsening of memory and other cognitive functions; no disturbance of consciousness; onset between ages 40 and 90, usually after age 65; and absence of other identifiable causes.

The diagnosis of *possible* Alzheimer's disease may be used when there are other significant diseases present but, on clinical judgment, Alzheimer's disease is considered the most likely cause of the dementia or when the presentation or course is somewhat unusual.

Histopathologic confirmation, based on postmortem examination of brain tissues, is required for the diagnosis of *definite* Alzheimer's disease.

Distinguishing between dementia and delirium is perhaps the most crucial differential diagnosis to make, because delirium can be rapidly fatal. Yet, if the cause of the delirium is treated, the patient may recover completely. Moreover, delirium may be superimposed on and aggravate the symptoms of an early or mild dementia; if the delirium is caused by drugs, intercurrent illness, or trauma, for example, treating the cause of the delirium may restore the patient's previous level of functioning.

Diagnostic Criteria for Delirium

When the DSM-III diagnostic criteria for delirium are considered, it becomes clear that they overlap considerably with criteria for dementia. The *first criterion* is, as mentioned earlier, clouding of consciousness, with reduced awareness of the environment and an inability to sustain attention to what goes on in the environment.

The *second criterion* is fulfilled by the presence of any two of the following four symptoms: (a) perceptual disturbances, such as misinterpretations, illusions, or hallucinations; (b) speech that is sometimes, but not always, incoherent; (c) disturbance of the sleep-wakefulness cycle, with insomnia and daytime drowsiness not uncommon; and (d) increased or decreased psychomotor activity.

Patients with dementia, who frequently wander and turn night into day, are very familiar to health care professionals largely because of the management problem they present; they also serve to emphasize the overlap between the criteria for dementia and delirium.

The *third criterion* for delirium is disorientation and memory impairment, which again we see in dementia.

The *fourth criterion,* however, is another one that distinguishes delirium from dementia: namely, that the clinical features usually develop within hours or days and tend to fluctuate over the course of the day. In dementia, we see a gradual onset over months or years, and fluctuations during the course of the day tend not to be so prominent.

Specific Treatments for Delirium and Dementia

Many causes of delirium and dementia have specific treatments. Dr. Phillip Henschke of Adelaide, Australia, proposed an acronym of the word dementia, which is helpful in organizing these causes:

Drugs. Frequently, we find a patient who is demented or delirious because of the inappropriate use of inappropriate drugs, the use of the wrong drug for a given patient, or the administration of a drug at the wrong time or in the wrong dosage.

Emotional disturbances, particularly depression, which may cause intellectual and memory impairment, can be difficult to distinguish from dementia. Many professionals make mistakes in this differentiation unless they are very careful and observe the patient over a period of time. Many of us feel that if there is the slightest doubt, we should treat the patient for depression because that is something we can cure in a significant percentage of patients.

Metabolic disturbances.

Endocrine disturbances, particularly thyroid disorders and diabetes.

Normal pressure hydrocephalus. It is not entirely clear which patients are the best candidates for surgery, but some improve markedly after surgery.

Trauma.

Infection or other illness.

Arteriosclerosis. Although the term is currently out of favor, some years from now someone may demonstrate how deposits in the small vessels of the brain have something to do with impaired circulation after all. Our teaching today, however, is that it is not deposits in the arteries, but the occurrence of small strokes which impairs mental functioning and causes dementia, so-called multi-infarct dementia. Current treatment is to reduce the tendency of the blood to clot and of platelets to aggregate. The efficacy of the treatment remains to be established, but for those who tolerate aspirin, it is certainly worth trying a baby aspirin every three or four days as a long-term preventive measure.

Making the Diagnosis of Alzheimer's Disease

With so many causes of delirium and dementia that are not causes of Alzheimer's disease, how do we make a diagnosis of Alzheimer's disease? First, we have to try to find out if the symptoms have a cause for which there is a specific treatment.

The most important source of information is the patient's medical *history*. Although getting a history from a patient who has problems with memory and language is very difficult, a great deal of information can be obtained if the patient is not too far advanced in the course of the disease or has a fluctuating state of consciousness. In addition, it is essential to get information from another person who knows the patient well. In cases where the patient has lived alone and has been secluded from other people, an informant may not be available. In such cases the diagnosis can be exceedingly difficult.

The second step in diagnosis is the *psychiatric evaluation,* including a careful mental status evaluation. We try to find out what the patient knows and does not know, what the patient can do and cannot do. Next to the history, this information provides the most important clues to diagnosis.

The third step is a careful *medical evaluation,* including a neurological examination and routine laboratory tests. The symptoms of Alzheimer's disease are mental and behavioral, so we try to rule out medical, including neurological, causes for the observed mental and behavioral symptoms.

There are a number of sophisticated *laboratory techniques* that may be helpful in diagnosis, but all current technologies have limitations. Both computerized tomography (CT) scans and magnetic resonance imaging (MRI) reveal the structure of the brain by looking at slices of the head as if it were being dissected. This enables us to localize special areas in the brain showing abnormalities, such as tumors or blood clots, that may be amenable to treatment. Typically, with Alzheimer's patients, CT scans show cortical atrophy with enlargement of the ventricles and sulci. However, the same degree of enlargement can be found in individuals who show no cognitive impairment. Hence, a CT scan cannot be used by itself to make a diagnosis of Alzheimer's disease, although it may help in identifying other causes of impairment.

Positron emission tomography (PET) scans show us the brain at work. Radioactively labeled deoxyglucose injected into the patient is metabolized by the brain and makes visible active parts of the brain. PET scans of Alzheimer's patients are mostly dark, indicating that little activity is going on in the brain, in marked contrast to the brightness shown by the active brain of a normal individual. Early in the disease, the temporal and parietal cortex show the most prominent deficits. PET scans are extremely expensive, however, and currently are used as a research tool rather than a clinical test.

Single photon emission computerized tomography (SPECT)

shows us the blood flow through the brain, rather than the rate of brain metabolism. This technique is likely to become clinically feasible and, when more fully developed, should be helpful in diagnosis. Again, however, no matter how sophisticated the technique, no single test can make the diagnosis of Alzheimer's disease.

Given the array of techniques available for the diagnosis of Alzheimer's disease, why is it so difficult for us to make the diagnosis? Five explanations come to mind.

First, the early symptoms vary. Although most people have memory impairment as their first complaint, others have major difficulty in expressing themselves. They cannot find the name for something (anomia), or they know exactly what they want to say but cannot say it (expressive aphasia). Other patients show irritability, while still others begin to have difficulty in manipulating objects. There is no single early symptom that signals the onset of the disease.

Second, the course of the disease may vary. It used to be held that a patient deteriorates rapidly and dies within 6 to 18 months; now we know that some patients live for 5, 10, even 20 years. We are not able to predict which patients will deteriorate rapidly and which will not. In addition, we used to think that if a patient showed no change in condition over a period of a year or so, our diagnosis must have been in error; we now know that patients may remain at a relative plateau for up to two years, if not longer.

Third, many symptoms of Alzheimer's disease are exaggerations of the changes manifested by older persons without dementia. This does not mean that the disease is the result of aging; most of us will not develop it even if we live to reach the century mark. We are, however, familiar with the experience of not being able to remember someone's name, only to have it come to mind minutes later. The difference between this phenomenon and the anomia shown by some Alzheimer's patients seems to be a matter of degree.

Fourth, there is a resemblance between some symptoms of depression and of Alzheimer's disease—for example, apathy and depressed mood. Moreover, many Alzheimer's patients are depressed early in the disease. Therefore, the diagnoses are difficult to differentiate.

Finally, there are no biological tests that will make a firm diagnosis. No blood tests, electroencephalograms, X-rays, or even the sophisticated technologies mentioned earlier, are definitive.

The Search for a Specific Diagnostic Test

The search for biological markers is going on in several research centers, including our own. Specifically, we have been looking at the response to a temperature gradient of certain white blood cells—polymorphonuclear leukocytes (PMNs)—that fight infection in the body. We call this response the philothermal response—from philo, meaning love, and thermal, meaning heat. We prepare a cell suspension from an ordinary blood sample and expose it to a temperature gradient, with the colder side at 32 degrees centigrade and the warmer side at 42 degrees centigrade. After three hours' exposure, very few cells from the Alzheimer's patients have moved to the warmer zone, while close to one-third of the cells from normal controls have migrated. To index the rate of movement, we constructed a ratio by dividing the number of cells remaining in the colder region by the number of cells that had moved to warmer areas. This so-called R-ratio is low for normal controls and higher for Alzheimer's patients. The results for the first 18 Alzheimer's patients and 18 age- and sex-matched cognitively intact controls were striking. Using an R-ratio of 11 as the cutoff, all but two of the Alzheimer's patients were above, and all but two of the controls were below (Jarvik et al. 1982). This response has the potential of being developed into a diagnostic test, if it can be verified with larger numbers of individuals.

Meanwhile, we wanted to know why there is a difference between the white blood cells from Alzheimer's patients and those from normal controls (as well as multi-infarct and depressed patients whose responses were like those of the normals). There are some clues. Families of Alzheimer's patients have a high frequency of Down's syndrome (Heston 1976; Heyman et al. 1983). In addition, Down's syndrome patients who live beyond their thirties develop Alzheimer's-like changes in their brains (Jervis 1948; Burger and Vogel 1973; Whalley and Buckton 1979; Wisniewski et al. 1985). Down's syndrome is caused by a chromosomal abnormality, an extra chromosome No. 21. Flaws in certain cell constituents, called micro-tubules, interfere with cell division and could lead to chromosomal abnormalities. Several years ago, Dr. Leonard Heston proposed that a defect in the microtubules is the common link between Alzheimer's disease and Down's syndrome (Heston 1976; Heston and Mastri 1977). An intact microtubular system is also needed for cells to move in a certain direction. Following the lead suggested by this connection, we took a drug called colchicine, a specific microtubule poison, and added it to cells from normal people. We found that these normal cells treated with colchicine mimicked the response of the untreated cells from Alzheimer's patients. Further, the more colchicine we added, the higher the R-ratio became (Fu et al. 1986). We are now engaged in other research to pursue this lead.

Although we have learned a great deal about Alzheimer's disease, we still know far too little, and that is why we have so much trouble making the diagnosis. There is an additional reason, however; many of us really do not want to make the diagnosis. We are caught in a dilemma—the patient and family may need to know as soon as possible, but there seems to be no reason to rush into making the diagnosis if a patient is functioning reasonably well, since we can only offer that patient treatment of specific symptoms as they appear.

That is especially a problem early in the disease when diagnosis is in doubt. For example, I prefer to wait until the patient has symptoms we can trust, and there are many (Winograd and Jarvik 1986). We can treat depression. We can treat paranoid ideas, but we had better make sure that the ideas are truly paranoid and not justified by reality (e.g., that no one is actually stealing the patient's clothes). We treat these symptoms with drugs.

Although we all warn about the dangers of drugs, they are still a major treatment resource. When the right drug is used in the right amount for the right patient at the right time, it can control paranoid symptoms, relieve depression, and ameliorate day-night reversal. We give sleeping medication, in spite of the problems associated with doing so, when other approaches fail. Thus, we still practice the art of medicine even though we like to believe that we have a science of medicine. Indeed, for the Alzheimer's patient, we do not yet have a science of medicine, although I feel confident that we will have one—the question is when.

A story is told about Sir Alexander Fleming that illustrates why I am so confident that we will soon find a solution to the Alzheimer's mystery. Fleming talked about the time when he was a medical student. One day in bacteriology lab, he noticed that his agar plate showed black spots surrounded by clear halos. When he asked his instructor about it, he was criticized for his careless technique, which was responsible for contaminating his culture with mold. He was instructed to start all over again. Fleming mused later about how many others, from instructors to professors to hundreds of bacteriologists around the world, must have encountered examples of those black spots surrounded by clear zones. Yet one very obvious question apparently had not occurred to any of them: if mold could prevent the bacteria from growing in a plate, might it not also prevent bacteria from growing in a human being? At that time, as a student, it did not occur to Fleming either; he did his experiment over, as instructed.

It seems to me that this is a prime example of how extremely obtuse even intelligent people may be. I do not think we have evolved that much since 1914. I think probably we are just as obtuse today. We might have the answer to Alzheimer's disease even now, if we were but able to recognize it. Let us hope one of us will recognize it before too long.

References

American Psychiatric Association, Task Force on Nomenclature and Statistics. 1980. *Diagnostic and statistical manual of mental disorders* (DSM-III), 3d ed. Washington, DC: American Psychiatric Association.

Burger, P. C. and F. S. Vogel. 1973. The development of the pathologic changes of Alzheimer's disease and senile dementia in patients with Down's syndrome. *American Journal of Pathology* 73:457 - 476.

Fu, T. K., S. S. Matsuyama, J. O. Kessler, et al. 1986. Philothermal response, microtubules and dementia. *Neurobiology of Aging* 7:41 - 43.

Heston, L. L. 1976. Alzheimer's disease, trisomy 21, and myeloproliferative disorders: Association suggesting a genetic diathesis. *Science* 196:322 - 323.

Heston, L. L. and A. R. Mastri. 1977. The genetics of Alzheimer's disease: Associations with hematologic malignancy and Down's syndrome. *Archives of General Psychiatry* 34:976 - 981.

Heyman, A., W. E. Wilkinson, B. J. Hurwitz, et al. 1983. Alzheimer's disease: Genetic aspects and associated clinical disorders. *Annals of Neurology.* 4:507 - 515.

Jarvik, L. F., S. S. Matsuyama, J. O. Kessler, et al. 1982. Philothermal response of polymorphonuclear leukocytes in dementia of the Alzheimer type. *Neurobiology of Aging* 3:93 - 99.

Jervis, G. A. 1948. Early senile dementia in mongoloid idiocy. *American Journal of Psychiatry* 105:102 - 106.

McKhann, G., D. Drachman, M. Folstein, et al. 1984. Clinical diagnosis of Alzheimer's disease: Report of the NINCDS-ADRDA Work Group under the Auspices of DHHS Task Force on Alzheimer's disease. *Neurology* 34:939 - 944.

Whalley, L. J., and K. E. Buckton. 1979. Genetic factors in Alzheimer's disease. In *Alzheimer's Disease - Early Recognition of Potentially Reversible Deficits*, ed. by A. I. M. Glen and L. J. Whalley. New York: Churchill Livingstone.

Winograd, C. H., and L. F. Jarvik. 1986. Physician management of the dementia patient. *Journal of American Geriatrics Society* 34:295 - 308.

Wisniewski, K. E., M. Wisniewski, and G. Y. Wen. 1985. Occurrence of neuropathological changes and dementia of Alzheimer's disease in Down's syndrome. *Annals of Neurology* 17:278 - 282.

Chapter 4

Caring for the Alzheimer's Patient

Responding to a Changing Population

Jacob Reingold

Twenty-five years ago, the Board of Directors of The Hebrew Home for the Aged at Riverdale (HHAR) was grappling with the issue of whether to admit wheelchair-bound individuals. It was understood in 1960 that our residents would become increasingly frail during their tenure, but admitting individuals who were already infirm was then viewed as a dramatic change in institutional mission. The Home had consciously developed over four decades from an overnight shelter into a *home* for the aged. Long before "deinstitutionalizing the institution" became a popular theme, a stimulating, warm, nonthreatening, and secure environment was viewed as part of our mission, as integral to care.

Today, we are again struggling with institutional mission and philosophy. The difference is that in the 1980s, our focus is on admission criteria, the development of programs, staffing, and reimbursement for the individual with severe cognitive impairment. Is a skilled nursing facility (SNF) bed an SNF bed, regardless of its occupant, as the New York State Department of Health defines it? Or do we believe that intermediate care facility (ICF) beds or SNF beds for individuals with dementing illnesses are different? And does age still have relevance to the institution's admission criteria?

33

Let me briefly review the changes that have come about in facility resident populations and then offer options for institutional responses.

Two million people suffer from Alzheimer's disease, the major form of dementia. Probably eight million persons' lives are affected by the disease if one includes family members (Reifler and Larson 1985). Professionals recognize that even with biomedical advances, increased numbers of clinical trials, and growing research funds, there are still enormous needs for services within the long-term care system (Reifler and Larson 1985).

Long-term care facilities have always cared for individuals with serious cognitive impairments. What has changed is not the existence of a population with dementing illnesses but rather the proportion of individuals with those illnesses within our institutions.

Estimates of the presence of cognitive impairment among nursing home residents range from 30 to 80 percent. While these statistics vary with definition, three surveys are of interest:

1. The 1977 National Nursing Home Survey (U.S. National Center for Health Statistics) found almost 60 percent of residents to have chronic brain syndrome or senility without psychosis.

2. A 1985 (Rovner and Rabins) assessment of a Washington, D.C., nursing home by Johns Hopkins Medical Center indicated that 70 to 80 percent of the residents had some form of cognitive disorder, of which Alzheimer's disease and multi-infarct dementia were the most common causes.

3. A 1984 survey of 42 skilled nursing facilities in upstate New York confirmed that 64 percent of the population had moderate to severe behavioral problems ranging from impaired judgment to danger to oneself and others (Zimmer et al. 1984).

Causes of Change

Why have nursing homes become the major source of institutional care for the mentally impaired population? Perhaps the primary reason is the deinstitutionalization of state mental hospital systems which paralleled the quadrupling of nursing home beds in the United States over the past 20 years (U.S. National Center for Health Statistics 1979; Johnson and Grant 1985; Brody et al. 1984).

The institutional long-term care system emerged as a major health care deliverer in the 1960s with the passage of Medicare, Medicaid, and Hill-Burton financing. ICFs were also developed by federal regulation in 1967. Note that this level of care now serves a much sicker population than was originally anticipated (Dunlop 1979). Changes in contemporary society from the demographic as well as nuclear family perspective have also increased the role of the nursing home; "the greying of America" relates most critically to the old-old age cohort as regards the implications for care. Concomitant with this population's growth is a decline in the availability of informal supports, due in part to changes as women seek employment, as families have fewer children, as family members live far apart, and as the divorce rate increases (Grossman et al. 1985; Brody et al. 1984; Johnson and Grant 1985).

The notion of a continuum of care, discussed as early as 1960, has catalyzed at least the conceptualization and often the availability and coordination of community services. The availability of community-based services is uneven, but where they exist, such services do increase an aging individual's ability to remain in the community. Hence, those entering a nursing home have become those who are more frail.

In a recent evaluation of nursing home admissions in New York, Katzman (1985) noted that 75 percent had some form of dementia upon admission; the symptoms did not develop following prolonged nursing home residency. While diagnostic abilities and protocols have improved, the medical community suggests that we have *not* reached the point of overdiagnosis. This is consistent both with our own experiences and with the literature which emphasizes that mental dysfunction is a leading cause of institutionalization (Johnson and Grant 1985). Further, we note that cognitive abilities and the availability of family supports differentiate between those who can be maintained at home and those requiring institutional supports (White

House Conference 1981; Weiner et al. 1980). Finally, public recognition that the nursing home is a viable, important element within the continuum of care, especially for Alzheimer's disease patients and their families, has increased substantially.

For many reasons—economics, the overwhelming burden of a 24-hour day, social disruptions—individuals with Alzheimer's disease are the least likely of the frail aged to be successfully maintained in the community (Brody et al. 1984). Haycox (1980) suggests that admission should be considered in the best interests both of the individual with dementia and of the family when the patient can no longer recognize the caregiver.

As we know all too well, once admitted to a nursing home, individuals with dementia, regardless of specific type, are unlikely to be discharged and usually will spend down to Medicaid eligibility levels. These individuals are often the long-term residents of nursing homes (Brody et al. 1984). This lengthy tenure is one of the inevitable results of improvement in our health care system.

Responses to Changing Needs

Given these realities, how do we assure that our institutions—continuing care facilities as well as discrete SNF/ICF programs—are congruent with the changed needs of our communities? Dependent upon institutional mission and goals, a variety of responses to the needs of the Alzheimer's patient and the family is possible, from denying admission to the patient, which regrettably still is practiced today, to establishing a range of nursing-home-centered services for the dementia patient.

I will first review the options that facilities have for dealing with Alzheimer's patients and then follow with a summary of a recent survey of AAHA members and the options they chose. The survey was funded by The Brookdale Foundation.

Option 1. *Exclude dementia or cognitive impairment from the criteria for new admissions.*

Even if a facility denies admission to new dementia patients, the current resident population will develop dementing symptoms. In that event, one of two courses can be followed:

- patients can be retained regardless of the degree of dementia developed, or

- patients can be discharged if their dementia poses management problems.

Option 2. *Develop selective admission criteria, based upon:*

- level of impairment
- age
- source of payment
- requirement of a special companion or aide.

Option 3. *Decide on placement within the institution and provision of special programs, services, or units:*

- provide no special care unit and no special programs for individuals with dementia;

- place individual patients throughout the facility and develop special programs. The placement may or may not be based upon functional assessments and progressive patient care; or

- develop special programs and establish special care units for homogeneous patient placement.

Option 4. *If admission to special care units is developed:*

- give priority to the current resident population;

- establish admission and discharge criteria so that when an individual no longer benefits from the therapeutic programs on the special care unit or requires additional or different medical care, he or she may be discharged to a more traditional SNF unit; or

- develop graduated special care units with progressive placement among the units.

Through earlier AAHA and North American Association of Jewish Homes and Services for the Aging (NAJHA) surveys and mailings, 26 facilities indicated that they have special programs for their dementia patients. Of these, 21 (81 percent) responded to the more in-depth questionnaire administered by HHAR in 1985. While more than 8,200 beds are represented by these facilities, this information is descriptive and presented with the caveat that these are self-selected facilities.

Placement decisions/special care units

- Fifteen facilities (71 percent) have discrete, planned, and designated special care units for individuals with dementia.

- Three facilities (24 percent) are considering development of such a unit(s).

- Two facilities (10 percent) are satisfied with the patient mix, using progressive, functional placement.

- One facility (5 percent) closed a behavioral problem unit in favor of heterogeneous placement.

Level of care

Within the facilities with special units, three have units at the ICF level. The remainder are SNF or are located in facilities offering only one level of care.

Number of beds

- The number of beds allocated to special care units ranges from 11 to 200 beds and from 6 to 51 percent of institutional bed complement.

- The average designation is 26 percent of bed complement or two such units in the facility.

There is a striking discrepancy between the fact that 26 percent of the beds are designated for patients with dementia and the fact that probably 50 percent of the patients have dementia.

Admission/discharge criteria

- Ten facilities (48 percent) give priority to in-house transfers for admission to a special care unit.

- Two facilities (10 percent) waive the 60 to 65-year admission criteria.

- Three facilities (14 percent) offer multiple special care units wherein placement is progressive between units.

- Eight facilities (38 percent) discharge patients from their units who are unable to benefit from programs, have physical care needs, or pose a danger to others.

Conversion/years open

- Nine facilities (43 percent) developed special care units through conversion of traditional ICF/SNF units.

- The oldest unit was established 20 years ago; one facility planned to open a unit soon.

- The average unit was six years old.

Continuum of care

Eight facilities (38 percent) extend services beyond institutional care for patients with dementia:

- Seven offer adult day care (health).
- Six undertake research.
- Two provide home health/home care.
- Two have outreach programs.
- One has a family support group.
- One offers case management.

Costs

- Nine facilities indicated their special care rate is the same as traditional SNF/ICF rates; however, two-thirds of those noted increased costs for such special services.

- The private rate varies from $40 to $120 per day.

No Right Answers

Efforts to respond to the needs of dementia patients and their families must reflect an institution's mission and philosophy, the need of its constituencies, reimbursement restrictions, regulatory constraints, and an institution's perception of balance.

For example, how does a facility provide a balanced environment in which the alert ICF resident can thrive and the demented SNF patient can be secure? While I cannot speak for every institution, it is my belief that placement by level of function, whether within a special care unit or through other forms of progressive patient placement, is the most advantageous approach for patients, families, staff, and the economic stability of the home.

The issue of homogeneous versus heterogeneous placement of individuals with dementia has been intellectually discussed in the literature. However, there has been little rigorous research as to its relative benefits.

Integration

It has been suggested that patients with varying levels of clinical need should be integrated on the same unit, that is, mainstreamed (Ablowitz 1983). It is further postulated that such integration is beneficial for all patients in the integrated unit. Those with lower levels of need may enjoy and benefit from helping the more impaired patients. Those who are more impaired may benefit from the companionship of a patient who functions on a healthier level.

Berman (1983) suggests that residents with different abilities compensate for fellow patients' lack of ability, seemingly without peer or staff pressure. Gurland et al. (1985) further suggest that staff and family resort to segregation when disconcerted by disruptive behavior.

Segregation

In contrast, Bowker (1982) reported strong evidence that mixing of patients with different levels of functioning may result in a sense of dehumanization. Specifically, such integrating of patients with substantial mental impairment may have a demoralizing impact upon those less impaired who need to prove their mental competency (Smithers 1977). Further, the severely impaired patient's response to a typical skilled nursing unit may be explosive or, in a setting that is too demanding, withdrawn. On the other hand, an oriented, rational individual may find a supportive, environmentally modified unit confining, too circumscribed, and devoid of interest (Goldfarb 1973).

An experiment on the effects of segregating and integrating the mentally impaired (Kahana et al. 1970) was inconclusive but did indicate the effectiveness of staff stimulation and attitude training. Experiences at both the Philadelphia Geriatric Center and The Hebrew Home for the Aged at Riverdale (Brody 1981 and Grossman et al. 1985) underscore the success of segregated areas within the facility for those who are extremely confused or whose behavior is severely disordered.

Other Questions

Beyond the establishment of special care units or special programming, there are other serious questions for facilities to assess when considering the care of patients with Alzheimer's disease.

- *Psychiatric support*: How is the balance between the medical model and the social components of care actualized? Are there adequate psychiatric supports available for assessment, treatment recommendations, participation in unit rounds, inservice, and multidisciplinary team planning?

- *Diagnosis*: Does the institution have a clinical protocol for the diagnosis of dementia? Have the intake department's psychosocial and medical procedures been updated to assure the availability of accurate information?

- *Design*: What kind of environmental adaptations are necessary to assure an environment that is pleasant, secure, and appropriately stimulating?

- *Family involvement*: Do institutional family groups include adequate educational and emotional supports for those persons related to Alzheimer's disease patients?

- *Staff involvement*: Have staff members, including the aides, been involved in the planning for special programming? Is there administrative support and sanction for regular staff support groups?

- *Community relations:* Has the facility assured that community-based services do not deny offerings to individuals with Alzheimer's disease?

Conclusion

We have reached a crisis in our institutions' ability to care for individuals with dementia and their families. While not a self-inflicted crisis, it nonetheless reflects a national inability to plan accurately for the future. But if we view *crisis* as the Chinese do, as a word formed from two characters meaning *danger* and *opportunity,* we can respond to the situation with intellectual stimulation and the emotional recognition that it is our obligation to design programs and services to alleviate the effects of this insidious disease which "robs victims of their minds and breaks the hearts and souls of families" (Aronson 1984).

Philosophy of Care

Daniel Sands

Dignity of the Person

Dementing illnesses such as Alzheimer's disease do not in some way obliterate the person. They do limit with progressive severity a person's ability to share life experiences and to respond to family members and others when they share their life experiences.

The stresses and strains experienced by caregivers apparently go unnoticed by the patient (Reifler et al. 1981). On the other hand, the patient's experiences of losing cognitive abilities, emotional stability, and social contact are locked inside, leaving caregivers to guess at what their loved one is thinking and feeling.

This limit on the ability to share interpersonally is probably central in leading some to the conclusion that a person afflicted with one of these diseases is no longer there or has ceased to exist as the individual he or she once was.

This is a philosophical and a theological assumption. There are no scientific data available to address whether the person is still in some fundamental sense existing as the self or what the quality or value of that existence is. Emil Brunner (1952), a Swiss theologian, offered the following thoughts:

> "True humanity is not genius but love, that love which man does not possess from or in himself but which he receives from God, who is love. True humanity does not spring from the full development of the intellect, but it arises through the reception, the perception, and the acceptance of the love of God."

Caregivers, who have a day-to-day vantage point, are impressed by the enduring richness of individual differences and by the still unique contributions that each patient makes to the community. A basic need for the Alzheimer's patient is recognition.

Normalization of Life

Normalization of life occurs when the social and physical environment still makes demands and offers choices so that the afflicted person is offered some challenge and the opportunity to find meaning through activity. The opportunity to maintain some degree of control, both perceived and actual, is a key clinical issue (Langer and Rodin 1976; Schultz 1976; Sands 1978; Suzuki and Harriss 1984). Research has shown that persons who perceive themselves in control do better cognitively, emotionally, and socially. Research has also shown that perceived control is closely related to the actual control experienced (Suzuki and Harriss 1984).

The cognitive limits imposed by Alzheimer's disease make it progressively more difficult for an afflicted person to interact with the environment. As the person begins to be unable to drive a car, manage a checkbook, or maintain a household, others in the environment are drawn in to assume those responsibilities.

Sometimes other persons will assume responsibility in such a way that excess disability is created. That is, caregivers begin to do things for the patient that he or she could still manage to do (Strauss and Glaser 1975). Of course, the opposite tendency is also likely; caregivers will expect patients to carry out functions that they are incapable of fulfilling.

In a situation where excess disability is a high potential event and where actual abilities are declining, a continuous assessment of an afflicted person's maximum degree of independence is required to maintain a proper approach to caregiving.

Clinical Implications: At Home or in a Home

Caregivers and patients tend to choose to maintain a common life space. Remaining in a home setting with family is most often the optimum state of affairs in terms of the person's dignity and normalization of life. Therefore, the sustaining familial caregiving system is of primary importance.

Providing family members with a break through day care and the opportunity to resume activities that have sustained them in the past (golf, club meetings, church, shopping, work, and so on) supports them in their caregiving.

Providing afflicted persons with opportunities to be out and about in an environment that makes demands on abilities and gives them an opportunity to be useful to themselves and others sustains them cognitively and emotionally and in some cases brings improvement.

In most cases, at some point the family is no longer able to sustain home care. If this occurs at the point where ambulation is no longer possible for the patient, then nursing home care or home care with appropriate assistance from a home health agency is appropriate.

If the family is no longer able to sustain home care and the person is still ambulatory and relatively healthy apart from the dementia, placement in a small board and care home for assisted living with 24-hour help at hand is recommended. In a six-bed assisted living facility the person is still continuously known to the staff. The staff may remain unknown to the patient by name due to memory failure. Patients are living in an environment they recognize as a house and in some cases identify as home, and still are able to maintain involvement in day care as an outside activity. The primary care focus in this continuum remains the patient's need for structure, recognition, and reorientation to the situation. The bottom line here is maintaining the patient in the least restrictive setting possible.

This philosophy of care assumes that we who are caregivers benefit from sharing in the lives of the patients and their families. In the most obvious way families and patients are our customers and are therefore the heart of our being here. In another sense they teach us how to do the things we do. Through a sometimes painful and sometimes humorous process of trial and error, we learn from patients how to operate a therapeutic milieu. Further, families and patients are teaching us something about ourselves as people: namely, that above all, human suffering is difficult but not without meaning or value. Neither is it something to be ashamed of or to be hidden away.

Principles for the Health Care Team

Herbert R. Karp

Physicians and other health care personnel concerned with the continuing care of persons with dementing illnesses are in a unique position to alleviate the devastating effect of these diseases. Recent advances in understanding degenerative, dementing illnesses such as Alzheimer's disease provide guiding principles for care. In addition, health professionals have the responsibility to practice these precepts in an ethical and humane manner.

Uppermost is the dictum that although the primary disease may be considered progressive and incurable, there is usually some aspect of the illness that can be modified to benefit not only the patient, but also the family and others concerned with the patient's welfare. Other guiding principles in caring for the demented patient follow.

Physical vulnerability. The brain, when affected by any generalized process, is more vulnerable to metabolic changes and toxins that can significantly alter brain function and patient behavior. It is therefore crucial to be attentive both to maintain adequate respiratory function, cardiac output, fluid, and electrolyte balance, and also to detect coexisting infection or other causes of fever.

Problems of perception. The demented patient virtually always has problems with perception and is therefore prone to confusion and agitation when in a strange or altered environment. Extrinsic factors, such as reduced lighting or heightened noise levels, and intrinsic factors, such as defects in hearing and vision, also interfere with perception and affect behavior. Patients are managed best in a familiar environment with familiar personnel. Facilities for these patients should:

- Employ furniture or other items from the patient's home to create a less threatening environment.

- Recruit a member of the family to be with the patient in periods of acute agitation.

- Increase the illumination in the patient's room, a small change that is always helpful.

- Attend to coexisting visual or hearing problems. Though the patient may be quite demented, his or her behavior can often be dramatically improved.

- Keep staffing as close as possible to a one-on-one ratio rather than assigning different persons to the various aspects of the patient's care, a method that exacerbates confusion.

Sedatives. The effects of sedatives, tranquilizers, and antidepressant drugs on a diseased brain are unpredictable and often paradoxical. Such medications may be needed, but they should be used with extreme caution. As a general rule, when a demented patient has an acute change in behavior, all drugs must be suspect. A demented patient is best managed in a facility that tolerates altered behavior rather than turning immediately to restraints or behavior-modifying medication.

Drug interaction. Any aging patient, and particularly any demented patient, who requires drugs for management of coexisting medical conditions presents special problems with regard to drug interaction. Therefore, periodic reviews by the physician in conjunction with a clinical pharmacist are mandatory.

Depression. Patients in all stages of dementing illnesses are frequently aware that their intellectual function is failing. This awareness can lead to profound depression and withdrawal, resulting in further limitations. Counseling of the patient, the family, and associates, particularly in the early stages of dementia, can lead to restructuring of the patient's pattern of daily living so that fewer demands are made on failing mental function. Antidepressants may be helpful, particularly those preparations with relatively low anti-cholinergic activity.

Family care. In the course of extensive evaluation of the patient, the family is frequently disregarded. Not only do members have needs that must be met by the attending team of caregivers, but they also are an invaluable source of information that can contribute significantly to the planning of the patient's continuing care and management.

Evaluate the family with the same systematic analysis used to evaluate the patient. As suggested by Dr. Dan Blazer of the Section of Geriatric Psychiatry at Duke University, much can be learned from the nature of the interactions between the family and the patient. Not only should the frequency of the interactions be noted, but also their quality. Blazer has identified several types of family interaction:

- compatible vs. conflictual
- cohesive vs. fragmentary
- productive vs. nonproductive
- fragile vs. stable
- rigid vs. flexible.

The atmosphere of the interaction between family and patient can be either relaxed or tense, hopeful or resigned.

Based on this approach, family members may reveal characteristic patterns of involvement:

- The *caretaker* can be depended upon to provide effective, objective, yet humane support to the patient and other family members.

- The *manager*, though not likely to provide the support himself or herself, is capable of organizing the family for support.

- The *victim* is more concerned with the effect of the illness on himself or herself than with the patient or other family members.

- The *facilitator*, wittingly or otherwise, creates situations leading to conflict.

- The *escapee* refuses to accept the reality of the patient's illness and its effects on the family.

Family members vary in their tolerance of disturbed behavior and in the degree to which they seek to influence, if not direct, the control of a patient's altered behavior even when the patient is receiving professional care in a skilled nursing or long-term care facility. This is not to imply, however, that the family should not be fully informed of the rationale for these types of decisions in patient management.

Just as the pattern of the patient's illness is constantly changing, so does the pattern of family structure and involvement. Hence, the health professional involved in the care of the demented patient must not lose the opportunity to make continued observations of family interactions and to apply them to the plan of management.

A cardinal family need is for a realistic and current assessment of the patient's illness. Only then can the family make definitive plans and be effectively supportive. Despite the difficulty in making a definitive diagnosis of Alzheimer's disease during life, a diagnosis can be made much more precise by careful, continued observation of the patient. The long-term care physician must be alert to clinical events that might suggest an alternative diagnosis, a superimposed illness, or further support for the impression of Alzheimer's disease.

The physician as team member. The physician concerned with continuing care of the demented patient, possibly more than in any other clinical circumstance, must participate in the care team as an active, contributing member, accepting comments from all members of the team whether or not they are considered to be health care professionals. As an example, a person from housekeeping may have made observations to which higher level personnel are not privy or which they have failed to notice. There must be a mechanism whereby such data can be received and incorporated into the process of planning care.

Similarly, although the care team may appear to be dominated by nonphysician personnel, the physician must be sensitive to the fact that his or her attitude toward the patient has a profound effect on the attitude of the rest of the team.

The physician as advisor. The patient or the patient's family will often turn to the physician for advice and counsel in matters that the physician might not consider to be within the purview of the medical profession. The physician may be called on to mediate or mitigate the political, social, and economic pressures that affect the demented patient's health care. Since demented patients (and often their families) are incapable of being their own advocates, the physician must be prepared to fill that role and to do so effectively. Problems often arise as the result of the uncritical application of cost-benefit and cost-effectiveness principles to decisions in health care; to paraphrase the medical economist, Rashi Fein: we must keep in mind that we live in a society and not in an economy.

In a discussion of ethical and humanistic considerations in care for the elderly, Steven Levenson (1983) reminds the health professional that one of the duties to the elderly patient is to recall that:

> Illness in any person represents a condition of exceptional vulnerability. Health is an essential requisite to freedom of choice and action. Illness is an assault on a person's very being—a force which erodes one's self-image. Thus, the older person is among the most vulnerable of all human beings. It is hard to envision treating disease in such a person without giving thought to the wounded humanity underlying the illness.

Levenson's admonition is particularly pertinent to the demented patient.

Organization of Services

Charles M. Gaitz and Nancy L. Wilson

Dementia is now recognized as a process that affects not only the individual victim but other family members as well. The provision of services must focus on the patient and the family as the unit of service. Individuals with dementia experience the illness and the changes it brings in unique ways. Likewise, family members who assume caregiving responsibility for dementia victims react to the disease process and their caregiving duties in highly individual ways (Rabins et al. 1982). Consequently, the types and amount of formal assistance needed by any one family or groups of families in a community will be highly individual.

Individuals with dementia are one subgroup of older people who have chronic functional limitations requiring them to receive one or more services on a sustained basis. Brody has outlined the ideal continuum of long-term support services that may be needed over time by disabled elders and their families. (See Figure 1.) (Brody and Masciocchi 1980). Due to prevailing social and health policy, many services in the ideal continuum are lacking for some or all of the impaired elders residing in a particular community. For example, in most states there is no public financing for any form of respite care, identified as the highest priority service need of caregivers of dementia patients (Morscheck 1986). Financing for long-term care continues to be heavily biased toward institutional responses and does not include adequate support for health and social service needs of community-dwelling elders, including those with dementia.

A discussion of the organization of services for dementia patients must consider a range of parameters, both individually and as they interact. Several principles of organization should characterize the delivery of services to patients with dementia. In particular, services should be coherent, comprehensive, and delivered by a multidisciplinary team (E. Brody 1981). Community agencies, residential facilities, and institutionally based services should have knowledgeable staff who are able to focus on patient and family needs.

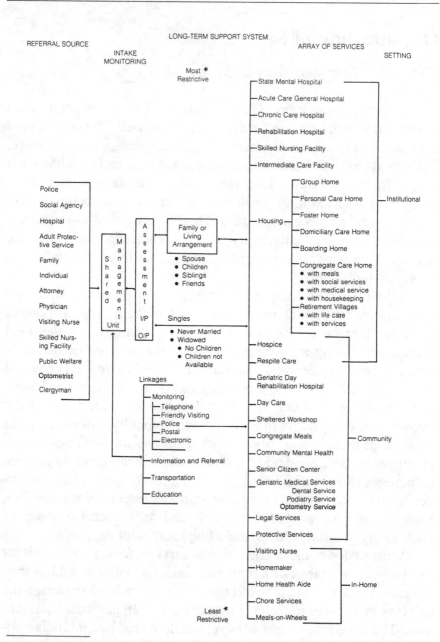

* The classification of from most to least restrictive is a general view of services and may vary within each service.

Figure 1. Inventory of Recommended Available Services, Appropriate to a Long-Term Care/Support System. Reprinted by permission of American Journal of Public Health 70(11) from S.J. Brody and C. Masciocchi. 1980. Data for long-term care planning by health systems agencies.

Comprehensive Care

Elderly patients are likely to have multiple problems. A thorough diagnostic evaluation will usually reveal a combination of physical, psychological, and social problems that contribute to their impairment. The interaction of these stresses is almost a prototype for the development of psychosomatic disorders. A few of the stresses and strains are indeed related to chronological age, but, as is true for persons of any age, successful treatment depends on resolving emotional as well as physical problems.

For a patient with dementia, a comprehensive treatment plan will take into account the full range of the patient's problems including the assets and liabilities of the patient's home or other living environment, the characteristics of patient and family, and the family's financial situation (Miller and Cohen 1981).

Ideally, care providers should consider the implications and interactions of all these factors and organize the delivery of services to meet all needs of all patients. The goal is rarely achieved in practice. Those responsible for care and treatment make choices according to the relative importance of various factors in the lives of the patients and in the available resources of a particular service system.

Since there is no single continuum of care, care providers go through a process in which, for example, the decision about where a patient is to live depends on his or her health status, mobility, family support, and preference. Financial considerations may take precedence: a person might be able to remain at home but not be able to afford supervisory help, necessitating institutionalization. The almost endless variations of individual circumstances and needs are met in the complex matrix of health care delivery (Brody and Masciocchi 1980).

Interdisciplinary Team Care

Another system of care delivery is the interdisciplinary team approach. In a typical community, an interdisciplinary team may be reasonably well integrated, but the community in which resources and facilities are truly linked is a rarity.

Ideally, an interdisciplinary team should be under a single administration, but experience shows that a consortium of agencies and practitioners also can work well. However constituted administratively, the team needs a coordinator or case manager to overcome obstacles and barriers, to ensure that the team's treatment plans are implemented, and to serve as an advocate for the patient.

The size and membership of the team depends on the treatment site and on patient characteristics such as level of ambulation, cooperativeness, adequacy of family support, financial resources, and other factors. The team's effectiveness depends on many factors including the role and responsibilities team members establish for themselves, their respect for one another, and their knowledge about each member's abilities and limitations (Gaitz and Wilson 1985).

There is no single model for organization of team service delivery. Even within an institution, teams may be organized in different ways to render services to persons living elsewhere, or they may care only for their own patients.

In addition to the several continua of care—of services, places, and patient characteristics—another variable to consider is the characteristics of therapists with different training and personalities. Persons trained in various disciplines share some characteristics, but differ in others. Psychiatrists, social workers, physicians, occupational therapists, and others all share with their colleagues mutual training experiences and knowledge, but the diversity of application is almost infinite and may be a function of the therapist's personal style and values.

Service settings utilizing the team approach need to design their collaborative work in a manner accepted and understood by each member. For example, teams working with dementia patients need to consider the unique contributions of psychiatrists and psychologists in the areas of evaluation and behavioral management, as well as the skills of social workers and nurses in home care planning and family counseling.

Team Care

Patients with dementia represent a prototype of patients who need a continuum of services; who may be living at home or in an institution; and who have a multiplicity of social, psychological, and physical health problems.

There are differences in the severity of dementia. Researchers have attempted to classify stages of dementia to help physicians predict prognosis and prescribe treatment. Unlike cancer, however, dementia does not yet boast a widely accepted staging model based on quantitative validation data. For purposes of characterizing the progressive cognitive decline and supporting treatment, some schemas propose a three- or four-level classification of dementia stages, ranging from mild to severe (Reisberg 1983).

Some patients with mild symptoms have memory impairment but are able to cooperate when being treated for concurrent medical or surgical problems. Other patients with more severe symptoms, who may be extremely withdrawn or have disabilities such as aphasia, may not be able to perceive sensations accurately or to tell what they feel; they may be indifferent to signs of illness such as a skin rash, abdominal pain, or temperature elevation.

Care should be designed to fit the needs of each, with an emphasis on the patient's mental status. A demented person who has fallen, for example, needs close observation and examination to determine whether the fall has resulted in a fracture, is related to heart disease, or has caused further brain damage. Such a fall and its cause and effect have implications for staffing patterns if the patient is in an institution; if the patient is living at home, the accident normally will lead to new decisions about the patient's supervision. Patients with mild forms of dementia can take more responsibility than can severely demented ones for reporting signs and symptoms of illness.

For treatment purposes, the range of patient characteristics must be matched with a continuum of living arrangements, services, family supports, community resources, and other variables.

The interaction of mental and physical status of demented persons is particularly important in planning care. Compliance with a medical regimen depends on a patient's ability to comprehend what is expected. A demented person who is mobile presents a different clinical picture and has different needs from one who has had a stroke and is hemiplegic. A demented patient in an intensive care unit for treatment after a heart attack deserves special attention. Not surprisingly, demented patients present special problems when diagnostic procedures are undertaken. Explanation, reassurance, and other forms of support may take more time and require more repetition than the same procedures administered to other types of patients.

Facilities and Services

Despite the fact that they share a common diagnosis, demented persons have diverse needs. Family members and friends provide most of the care and support (E. Brody 1985); hence, formal services that focus on both patient and family needs are especially important. Due to burdensome responsibilities, nonprofessional caregivers of demented persons often display significant levels of stress and also physical and emotional problems. Caregiver support, education, and relief are provided in such programs as adult day care, respite care, and counseling (Zarit et al. 1980).

Depending on their needs and circumstances, patients with dementia may require continuous or intermittent supervision with some or all of their daily activities. Institutions and community-based agencies provide services that include meals, social activities, psychiatric treatment, and home maintenance, but most of these programs are not designed to deal with demented old people per se (E. Brody 1981). Even when they are prepared to serve persons who have physical, mental, and social impairments, the programs are likely to vary in emphasis, and patients with dementia may not receive as much attention as those who have other impairments. Cognitive impairment, for example, may be seen as a corollary of aging, and its importance as a factor in treatment may be given little or no attention. Approaches targeted to demented patients are few, and they may be inadequate for patients with health problems in addition to dementia.

Thus, programs serving the elderly may not be staffed adequately or targeted sharply enough to serve the special needs of demented persons. Rarely does one find a program or an agency that holds to the principle that comprehensive care requires attention to several parameters of care.

Agencies tend to adopt one system and ignore many other dimensions of service need. Recognition of the heterogeneity of the elderly has been achieved; society no longer believes that chronological age is an all-encompassing factor. Now it is time to give up the idea that elderly persons with dementia can be cared for by a system that addresses only one part of the problem.

Management of Fragmented Services

In most communities, the network of facilities and services to provide comprehensive care for elderly persons is incomplete, and the linkages among existing services are weak. At the same time and despite these inadequacies, rising public costs for health services and nursing home care have become an increasing concern.

One response to these problems has been the expansion of managed care models including social health maintenance organizations (Beatrice 1985). A service or case manager works with each older person to assess needs and arrange for appropriate care including services from multiple agencies if needed. Several community long-term care demonstration models have tested the effectiveness of structured case management and expanded in-home services for functionally impaired older people, including persons with dementia. The largest of these demonstrations was the Channeling Demonstration carried out in ten communities around the country (Baxter el al. 1983). None of the centers has analyzed the data comparing subgroups of patients with and without dementia. Meanwhile, the experimental results and programmatic findings of the various projects are best summarized as follows:

1. Eligibility for inclusion in the studies varied among centers. Some treated only patients who had met requirements

for nursing home placement. Others included patients who did not meet these criteria but were functionally impaired. Cost savings were demonstrated only for those centers that restricted their caseload to patients eligible for and seeking nursing home care (Capitman 1982).

2. No dramatic improvements in the client's physical and mental functioning were reported, but increased satisfaction and well-being were noted by clients who received case management services compared with those who did not have such assistance (Weissert 1985).

3. Anecdotal observations: Physically impaired clients living in the community were found to have, in addition, a variety of emotional and cognitive impairments. This was not unlike the experience reported by investigators of the mental status of persons residing in institutions, but, as we said before, the factor of mental status had not been given sufficient attention.

The results reported so far suggest that planning for comprehensive long-term care must include (Wilson 1983):

1. provision of mental health evaluation and service for all who need it by establishment of a continuum of inpatient and outpatient services. Currently, few people who require long-term care are being treated by mental health professionals.

2. training of service managers to deal with patients who have mental health problems, especially dementia.

3. training techniques for family members who provide long-term care to demented relatives; support for the family members who carry this extra burden.

Conclusion

Discussing the need for a full range of services to provide long-term care is common, but the full collaboration desired is rarely achieved. We overlook the mental health needs of persons who require long-term care; services for demented elderly persons are in particularly short supply.

Specific programs organized within larger services can give more attention to demented patients. Much can be done to alleviate the misery of these patients and the desperation of their families. Better staff training is of course essential, as are closer working relationships between practitioners and agencies that are part of the hoped-for continuum of care.

References

Ablowitz, M. 1983. Letter to the editor: Pairing rational and demented patients in long-term care facilities. *Journal of American Geriatric Society* 31 (10):627.

Aronson, M.D. 1984. Introduction. *Generations* 9:5 - 6.

Baxter, R., R. Applebaum, J. Callahan, et al. 1983. The planning and implementation of channeling: Early experiences of the National Long Term Care Demonstration. Princeton: Mathematica Policy Research.

Beatrice, D. F. 1985. Beyond institutional long-term care: Community care system. In Aging *2000: Our Health Care Destiny, Volume II: Psychosocial and Policy Issues,* ed. by C. M. Gaitz, G. Niederehe, and N. Wilson, 279 - 286. New York: Springer-Verlag.

Bergman, J. 1983. Mentally ill in nursing homes? Yes, if .... *Geriatric Nursing* 3:98 - 100.

Bowker, L. H. 1982. *Humanizing institutions for the aged.* Lexington, MA: Lexington Books.

_____. 1985. The informal support system and health of the

future aged. In *Aging 2000: Our Health Care Destiny, Volume II: Psychosocial and Policy Issues, e*d. by C. M. Gaitz, G. Niederehe, and N. Wilson, 173 - 190. New York: Springer-Verlag.

Brody, E.M., M. Lawton, and B. Leibowitz 1984. Senile dementia: Public policy and adequate institutional care. *American Journal of Public Health* 74(12):1381 - 1383.

Brody, S. J. and C. Masciocchi. 1980. Data for long-term care planning by health system agencies. *American Journal of Public Health* 70:1194 - 1198.

Brunner, Emil. 1952. The *Christian doctrine of creation and redemption*. Philadelphia: The Westminster Press, 58 - 59.

Capitman, John. 1982. *Preliminary report of work in progress*. Berkeley, CA: Berkeley Planning Associates.

Dunlop, B. D. 1979. *The growth of nursing home care*. Lexington, MA: Lexington Books.

Gaitz, C. M., and N. L. Wilson. 1985. Care of the elderly by interdisciplinary teams. Presentation for conference on "Recent Advances in Geriatric Care." Boston: Harvard Medical School.

Goldfarb, A. I. 1973. *Aged patients in long-term care facilities*. Rockville, MD: National Institute of Mental Health.

Grossman, H. D. et al. 1985. The milieu standard for care of dementia in a nursing home. *The Journal of Gerontological Social Work,* Fall issue.

Gurland, B. J., D. E. Wildner, and J. A. Toner. 1985. A model for multi-dimensional evaluation of disturbed behavior in the elderly. New York: Medical and Scientific Books.

Haycox, J. A. 1980. Occupational notes: Care of the demented patient, The question of nursing home placement. *The New England Journal of Medicine* 303(3):165 - 166.

Johnson, P. L., and L. A. Grant. 1985. *The Nursing Home in American Society*. Baltimore: The Johns Hopkins University Press.

Kahana, E., B. Kahana, and K. Jacobs. 1970. Functionally integrated therapy programs for the elderly. Presentation. Toronto: The Gerontological Society.

Katzman, R. 1985. Dementia in the context of the teaching nursing home. *The Teaching Nursing Home,* ed. by L. E. Schneider et al. New York: The Beverly Foundation, Raven Press.

Langer, E. J., and J. Rodin. 1976. The effects of choice and enhanced personal responsibility for the aged: A field experiment in an institutional setting. *Journal of Personality and Social Psychology* 34 (2):191 - 198.

S. A. Levenson. 1983. Ethical and humanistic considerations in the care of the elderly. In *Clinical Aspects of Aging*, 2d ed., ed. by W. Reichel, 522 - 532. Baltimore: Williams and Wilkins.

Miller, N. E., and G. D. Cohen, eds. 1981. *Clinical Aspects of Alzheimer's Disease and Senile Dementia*. New York: Raven Press.

Morscheck, P. 1984. An overview of Alzheimer's disease and long-term care. *Pride Institute Journal of Long-Term Health Care* 3(4):4 - 10.

Rabins, P. V., N. L. Mace, and J. J. Lucas. 1982. The impact of dementia on the family. *Journal of the American Medical Association* 248:333 - 335.

Reifler, B., et al. 1981. Problems of mentally ill elderly as perceived by patients, families, and clinicians. *Gerontologist* 21:165 - 170.

Reifler, B., and E. Larson. 1985. Alzheimer's disease and long-term care: The assessment of the patient. *Journal of Geriatric Psychiatry* 18(1):9 - 27.

Reisberg, B., ed. 1983. *Alzheimer's Disease*. New York: Free Press.

Rovner, W., and P. V. Rabins. 1985. Mental illness among nursing home patients. *Hospital and Community Psychiatry* 36(2):119 - 128.

Sands, D. 1978. The relationship of stress, blood pressure and focus of control to intellectual functioning in women over 65. Unpublished doctoral dissertation, Emory University, Atlanta, Georgia.

Schulz, R. 1976. Effects of control and predictability on the physical and psychological well-being of the institutionalized aged. *Journal of Personality and Social Psychology* 33(5):363 - 373.

Smithers, J. A. 1977. Institutional dimensions of senility. *Urban Life* 6(3):251 - 276.

Strauss, A. L., and B. G. Glaser. 1975. Chronic illness and the quality of life. St. Louis: C. V. Mosby Co.

Suzuki, T., and M. Harriss. 1984. Improvement in the social functioning of the cognitively impaired. Unpublished master's thesis, California State University, San Diego.

U.S. National Center for Health Statistics. 1979. Behavioral problems among patients in skilled nursing facilities. *Nursing Home Survey: 1977 Summary for the United States.* Washington, DC: NCHF, DHEW, PHS.

Weiner, A., M. Faletti, and B. Locke. 1980. *Statewide hospital discharge study: An assessment of factors impacting upon the discharge placement of elderly persons in the State of Florida.* Research report. Tallahassee, FL: Florida Department of Health and Rehabilitative Services.

Weissert, W. G. 1985. The cost effectiveness trap. *Generations* 9(4):47 - 50.

White House Conference on Aging. 1981. *Final Report.* Washington, DC: GPO.

Wilson, N. L. 1983. Serving impaired elders in the community: The interface of case management with mental health services. Presentation at the 36th annual meeting of the Gerontological Society of America.

Zarit, S., K. Reeves, and J. Bach-Peterson. 1980. Relatives of the impaired elderly: Correlates of feelings of burden. *Gerontologist* 20:649 - 655.

Zimmer, J. G., N. Watson, and A. Treat. 1984. Behavioral problems among patients in skilled nursing facilities. *American Journal of Public Health* 74(10):1118 - 1121.

Additional Reading

Gaitz, C. M. 1970. Obstacles in coordinating services for the care of the psychiatrically ill aged. *Journal of the American Geriatrics Society* 18:172 - 181.

_____. 1984. Dementia: Implications for patient care. In *Interdisciplinary Topics in Gerontology: Volume 20, Patient Care,* ed. by H. P. Von Hahn, 185 - 191. Basel: S. Karger.

Sands, D. 1983. Adult day care for Alzheimer's patients. *Gerontologist* 23(1):21 - 23.

Chapter 5

Case Studies of Care

Many Problems, Some Solutions: The Menni Unit

Hazel Mummah-Castillo

The Problem

The United States is marking the completion of the second decade since the implementation of the Medicare reimbursement system for the health care of its elderly. At Medicare's inception, the elderly and caregivers alike perceived this innovation as a godsend to the frail aged; institutional health care became available to large numbers who previously could not afford its cost.

Health caregivers, however, were soon to discover that along with its blessings came changes and problems of sometimes gargantuan proportions. The number of nursing home beds grew at a pace far more rapid than did the body of knowledge defining geriatric care. Administrators, nurses, physicians, and others became frustrated and discouraged as they attempted to deal with problems inherent to the mandatory use of the medical model for their patients, while the primary problem of more than 50 percent of these clients was dementia. Burnout, a term that became popular in the late 1970s, often succinctly described the state of nursing home personnel, while the media had a heyday describing long-term care atrocities such as overtranquilization or restraint of patients.

By the early 1980s, the problems that had seemed so murky in the 1970s were being identified, and solutions were beginning to appear. Journal articles and textbooks, for example, were describing the dementias: how to differentiate one from another and what to do for patients with these brain cell-destroying diseases.

It was during these exciting times that I was hired as a nurse-gerontologist consultant to assist the staff of St. John of God Nursing Hospital in creating a unit exclusively for the care of dementia patients.

St. John of God Nursing Hospital and Residence is a nonprofit 181-bed facility located in the heart of urban Los Angeles. While over 50 percent of our total population had some degree of dementing disease, the 18 of those patients who were ambulatory seemed to need disproportionate amounts of staff time, were losing weight, and were continually getting into safety-jeopardizing situations. Their tendencies to wander from our unlocked facility kept the entire staff anxious because they frequently succeeded! Incident reports describing their safety hazards were numerous. The fire department emergency squad was required once to free a gentleman's hand from an elevator door in which it was unbelievably entangled.

The nursing staff complained that these patients required too much time for care, were difficult to deal with, and did not respond to care delivery the way they "should have." Many of the families of these patients hovered about angrily, upset and uneasy; their concerns further encroached upon staff time and patience. Others simply stayed away.

We conducted a literature search in late 1982, in the hope of finding an existing care model to emulate in our nursing home, but we failed to locate one. The search did, however, bring to our attention a number of excellent journal articles and books. Descriptions of an appropriate environment, plus the help of a specialist in environmental design, prompted immediate planning to create a wandering garden with direct access from the dementia unit.

My first task was to assemble a steering committee to create the care concepts for the dementia unit. This committee included several of our staff physicians, the facility medical director, the administrative staff, representatives from the multidisciplinary staff throughout the house, and experts from our community. Throughout the planning process, we shared information and solicited advice from the nursing staff at all levels; we knew that if they did not feel a part of this innovation, it would never succeed.

Goals

One of the most difficult tasks of the steering committee was mutually to agree upon and establish goals. We were amazed to find that each of us had a personal impression of how this heretofore unseen unit would look and function and whom it would actually serve. After some difficulty, the steering committee finally agreed upon the following three goals.

- To enhance the well-being of each individual patient, we would modify the environment to provide maximum support, select and train a special staff to better understand the patient's needs, and seek to reverse any existing remediable condition causing the dementia.

- The caregiving model was to be an evolving prototype.

- We would disseminate information learned into the body of literature and into the community.

Criteria for Admission

To pinpoint and define the population to be served, the following admission criteria were established. The patient would have to:

- be ambulatory; use of devices such as canes and walkers would be acceptable.

- have a diagnosis of dementia such as Alzheimer's or multi-infarct dementia or symptoms which strongly suggested brain cell-damaging disease.

- be free from communicable disease.

- have a physician's order for admission.

- be determined by preadmission assessments to display behavior patterns that could be safely controlled within care capacities of the Menni Unit.

Within a relatively short time the steering committee had in place policies and procedures (including protocol guidelines for assessment of individual patients and medical records forms for gathering and clarifying patient data) that outlined the way in which the needs of our ambulatory dementia patients would be addressed. We spelled out strategies that we hoped would have an impact on the patients' care needs regarding safety, memory loss, communications, nutrition, and potential for disruption of the family unit. We did not address needs relating to the depression commonly seen in the earlier stages of dementia or to mobility as it is threatened in preterminal and terminal stages, because our unit's population consisted chiefly of persons with moderate to severe brain cell damage who were still ambulatory. The unit was named the Benedict Menni Unit to honor the memory of an earlier member of the owners' order, The Hospitaller Order of St. John of God; it is now affectionately called the Menni Unit.

Safety

The 22-bed physical design of the Menni Unit was structured to meet the safety needs of this specific group of patients. A large wandering garden, accessed freely from either end of the unit, transforms the pacing behaviors that had previously been viewed as irritating or dangerous into healthy physical exercise. A horticulturist made a careful selection of nonpoisonous plants to decorate the wandering garden. Staff task schedules include physical patrolling of the gardens every 15 minutes to monitor the safety of anyone utilizing the paths or seating. Areas of egress from the Menni Unit are protected by decorative garden fencing; only persons with intact cognition are able to release gate latches.

Refurbishing of the Menni Unit was accomplished under the direction of an environmental specialist who suggested numerous ways to modify the physical setting in order to increase the number of visual clues. For example, doorways and baseboards are painted a dark brown to contrast with lighter walls, thus enabling aged eyes to demarcate boundaries more clearly. Corners of the fireplace, shelves and cupboards, and dividers are rounded to minimize injury to patients who might strike against them during a fall. Medication carts, propelled through the halls for dispensing medications in other units, are replaced by a medication room located away from patient access. Housekeepers' carts keep poisonous cleaning materials in locked compartments. Personal grooming items, including razors, scissors, or harmful cosmetics are removed from patients' rooms; televisions and other electrical appliances are used only in areas where staff are in constant supervision. Doors to patients' rooms are kept closed when patients are occupied elsewhere. Patients are encouraged to join group activities or remain involved in independent behavior in areas where staff eyes may more efficiently monitor safety needs.

During the two years that the Menni Unit has been operational, alterations in the physical design, coupled with implementation of a psychosocial care model and a creative social activities program, have totally eliminated what used to be an awesome number of serious accidents involving this special group of patients.

Memory Disturbances and Communications

While our primary goal when planning the physical design of the Menni Unit was safety, we were also concerned about providing a physical environment capable of enhancing reality orientation and tranquility for patients, staff, and visitors. We made efforts to reduce the institutional ambiance and replace it with a homelike atmosphere capable of triggering memory and sensory stimuli. Clocks, calendars, and memory boards are plentiful. In each patient's bedroom unit there is a corkboard where relatives are encouraged to tape photographs, cards, and other items to clue memory connections with their own identity and the identities of significant others. These boards not only help the patient to remember his or her identity, but also provide valid information to staff members during conversations. Frequently, a mini-life review occurs as pictured events and people are discussed.

Other artifacts are welcomed in patient rooms or common areas. One patient has a worn teddy bear; his wife speculates that he perceives it as a beloved, little brown dog from his recent past. Another has a world championship boxing trophy (when we relate to the owner of this three-foot-high prize as "Champ," we always get an appropriate response); others have flowers or a faded piece of framed needlepoint. A pair of lovebirds screech at us from their cage in a sitting area; several of the patients watch their antics for long periods of time.

Since our patients have severe memory impairment, reality orientation as a formal therapeutic modality is effective for only three or four of them. We find reminiscing therapy, in both formal sessions and informal conversations, more helpful in retrieving old memories or improving current orientation. Pets and small children often visit during these sessions. It is not uncommon to be greeted at the door of the Menni Unit by the aroma of baking cakes. The ladies are heavily involved in cooking activities, and an occasional man will join them. Almost all of the patients get involved with sensory stimuli; feeling different textures, sniffing familiar odors, or touching an infant frequently can elicit responses even from persons whose communication skills are grossly damaged.

Most of the patients in the Menni Unit are to a marked degree aphasic; their language skills are usually impaired early in Alzheimer's disease, and by the time they are admitted to the Menni Unit they cannot remember how to address their own family members. The staff, chosen for patience and for nurturing personalities and given training to understand the nature of brain cell-damaging disease, seem to develop communication skills that transcend the need for articulate language skills. Bonding seems to take place between staff members and patients; frequently one of the caregivers will be able to interpret a particular patient's communicative gestures to those of us who spend less time in close contact with the patient. Communication involves smiles and touching; understanding appears easy and normal.

Aggressive behavior by these patients is so rare that when it does occur, staff members perceive it as unusual and often request a thorough assessment of the patient's physical and medical needs, explaining, "He 'acted out' this morning, so something must be wrong with him." The catastrophic reactions, described in literature as inappropriate responses to stimuli (a term coined by Goldfarb in the 1940s to describe inappropriate responses occurring when patients were pressed for memory performance), seem to occur in our patients only when they have concurrent pain-producing disease or other problems.

Nutrition

There is very little definitive information available regarding special nutritional needs of the dementia patient, but one frequently finds allusions in the literature to the inevitable weight loss in the patient with Alzheimer' s disease. A prime motivating factor in our search for improved care methods for the dementia patients at St. John of God Nursing Hospital was indeed their consistent pattern of weight loss.

Nutritional planning for the Menni Unit provides for an extra meal before bedtime plus nutrition breaks mid-morning and mid-afternoon.

Fully as important as the amount and quality of food intake is the demented patient's state of hydration. Maintaining adequate food balance requires careful monitoring; these patients are prime candidates for inadequate fluid intake because patients cannot remember how to use a drinking fountain, cannot express feelings of thirst, and are unable to remember the basic principles of hygiene to safeguard the cleanliness of water pitchers left at the bedside. To ensure adequate hydration, the daily care schedule provides numerous occasions for serving water and other beverages.

Meals are served in the common dining rooms. If a patient is temporarily ill and must have a meal at bedside, a nursing assistant remains with him/her to assist and monitor the process. Patients are reminded to stay in the dining room until all food is eaten, chew the food, swallow the food, and refrain from eating another person's servings. For patients who have difficulty swallowing, the food is cut, chopped, or pureed as necessary. Since the potential danger of choking is great, persons competent in first aid are always present and watchful at mealtime. Dining is treated as a socialization event; usually there is music, and dancing often precedes dinner.

Disruption of the Family Unit

Far from fulfilling the ugly stereotypes of Americans gladly abandoning their elderly to the care of nursing homes, the families of our Menni Unit patients usually demonstrate and express high levels of anxiety or concern as they consider admitting a demented patient to the Menni Unit. During preadmission interviews, they are given ample time to learn and understand the process, are encouraged to visit the unit frequently and without the presence of administrative personnel if they wish, and often are given information about the nature of the disease that is destroying the cognitive functions of their family member. When they perceive brain cell damage as a physical disease rather than a psychiatric disorder, they often become less distraught.

During the preadmission process, we ask the family to complete a History of Illness form for the medical record. This form not only seeks information that the physician requires for diagnosis, but also elicits information about the manner in which the family cared for the prospective patient in the home. This process has proved helpful because the physician need not uselessly press the patient for this information, the caregiving staff gets a preliminary understanding of the patient's needs and habits, and the family is assured of the value of its input regarding the continuum of care from home to institution. On the day of admission, the family assists in creating the patient's care plan.

Open visiting hours further serve to reassure the family. Many continue to visit daily while others do not. To make their visits comfortable, family members are encouraged to be active with the patient, perhaps escort the patient on a walk, eat lunch together, or mutually attend an activity or worship session. In this way, the pain generated by the loss of ability to interact on a highly cognitive level is minimized, and visits are perceived as satisfying.

Results of Care Pattern Changes

The problems that promoted the creation of the Menni Unit— safety, nutrition, memory deficits (that compound behavioral problems), communication, and family interactions—seem to have become greatly reduced in its two years of operation. In a search for more objective data, we sought some measure in the areas of safety, nutrition, and reduction in the use of psychotropic drugs. We focused on a group of 10 of the 18 original patients who had been housed in various units within the facility and for whom records existed for a period of at least six months prior to transfer to the Benedict Menni Unit. The data were recorded six months prior to the move to the unit in October of 1983 and then six months after the transfer. The mean age of this group was 81.7 and their medical records listed an average 4.4 diagnoses (including the one addressing the dementia). Three patients were transferred to a hospital for a short spell of acute care in the six months after admission to the Menni Unit. (Subject A had a major congestive heart failure episode and spent three weeks in a cardiac care unit; Subject G was diagnosed as having acute carcinoma in the abdomen; and Subject I had a thrombophlebitis in her leg). All are doing well at the current time (two years after transfer to the Menni Unit), with the exception of Subject G who is no longer ambulatory and is therefore a patient in another skilled unit now.

Figure 1 reveals that 9 of the 10 subjects had a gain in weight from April 1983 to April 1984. The average weight gain was 5.1 pounds.

To determine psychotropic drug usage, the number of dosage units of tranquilizers, antipsychotics, and sleeping medications actually given in a one-month period was measured in April 1983 and compared with dosage units actually given in April 1984. (The + or - refers to the number of dosage units given in April 1983 minus the April 1984 number.) The average decrease was 36.4 units.

Figure 1. Menni Unit Patients—Change Measures 4/83 to 4/84.

Subject	Age	Diag. #	Lbs. +/-	Drugs Doses +/-	Serious Episodes in Time Period
A	79	6	-14	-212	In ICU x 2 weeks; March 1984 (CHF)
B	71	3	+9	-0-	None
C	79	5	+9	-30	None
D	90	4	+8	-90	None
E	86	4	+8	- 1	None
F	88	4	+8	-0-	None
G	67	5	-2	+4	Active CA
H	73	6	+22	-59	None
I	87	3	+1	+24	Thrombophlebitis;4.84
J	87	4	+2	-0-	None
Averages	81.7	4.4	+5.1	-36.4	

A Therapeutic Environment at Morningside House

Cynthia J. Wallace

When Morningside House opened its doors in 1974, we had 147 skilled nursing and 239 health-related (intermediate care) residents. The facility, designed by Philip Johnson, is magnificent and was a perfect residential health care facility for the frail elderly.

In 1976, New York State implemented admission and placement criteria for long-term care facilities. The criteria included scoring resident assessments with regard to various activities of daily living, behavioral characteristics, mental acuity, and medical needs. For example, the need for some assistance with bathing had a score of 17, for total assistance with bathing a score of 24; occasional poor judgment scored 15. The resident had to have a score of at least 60 to be eligible for health-related nursing and a score of 180 to be eligible for skilled nursing.

Shortly after this system was implemented, it became apparent that a unique group of residents was being identified: those who scored about 150 points on this placement tool. Their placement score was too low for skilled nursing, but their mental impairment manifested by behavioral problems—wandering, and need for guidance, direction, and therapeutic intervention —rendered them inappropriate for the health-related level of care. There simply was not sufficient staff in health-related care to provide the structure and support that these residents required. Additionally, the healthier residents were most intolerant of aberrant behavior; they frequently ridiculed, embarrassed, and sometimes even assaulted the more impaired individuals.

Clearly, definitive administrative action had to be taken to resolve this dilemma. The administrative staff, primary caregivers, and representatives from all the therapies met to identify specific problems and to brainstorm about solutions. We concluded that a special unit to meet the unique needs of these residents was required. In those days, we did not speak of Alzheimer's disease; we called our unit a special unit for the ambulatory confused.

The unit was established and staffed as a health-related unit. The auxiliary staff were assigned and handpicked based on their ability to cope, their maturity, and their judgment. We were clear that our goal was not to create merely an environment in which therapy took place but a therapeutic environment, and we considered a loving, caring, compassionate staff as an essential component of that environment.

The various therapeutic disciplines created special programs for these residents. The programs were conducted on the unit, since transferring the residents to activities off the unit tended to pre-cipitate agitation and various other forms of aberrant behavior.

The unit functioned well as a health-related unit for about 12 months. Then, ever so slowly, evidence that all was not well began to show up. Staff members were experiencing difficulty in dealing with the gradual deterioration of the residents; the residents were more difficult to manage as their dementia progressed; families were anxious because their resident was failing; and we all realized that the staff as a whole was not coping well enough with the situation.

Again, administrative action was required; consequently we held meetings with all participants. The meetings concluded that ap-plication should be made to the state requesting that the unit be converted from health-related to skilled nursing and that the unit be dedicated to caring for residents with Alzheimer's disease and related disorders. The unit was staffed at the skilled nursing level, and the staff renewed efforts to develop programs designed to reduce epi-sodes of aberrant behavior and agitated outbursts.

Staff

Despite the administration's efforts to provide staff with the skills required to function in this unique setting, we were not doing enough. There was tension and uncertainty evident in the behavior of the staff. Residents frequently acted out. Families were anxious. We were not satisfied; we had not as yet created a therapeutic environment, and we were uncertain how to do so.

At this point, we sought help from an expert in the field, a psychologist whose expertise included staff training in specialized care for residents with dementia. In addition to training staff, the psychologist helped us develop a variety of multidisciplinary therapeutic interventions for residents depending on their degree of dementia. All staff—management, therapeutic, and support—were invited to the educational sessions. Primary caregivers on the Alzheimer's unit received additional educational programs.

Concurrently, the multidisciplinary team assessed all residents at Morningside House. Based on their needs as defined by this assessment, residents were placed in special therapeutic groups designed to be appropriate to each resident's degree of dementia. To the casual observer, the therapeutic group might look like recreational therapy—music and movement, reminiscence, or sensory stimulation. These groups have a definite goal, however, and meet for a specific number of sessions. The residents are reassessed at the conclusion of a full session and, based on the assessment, are assigned to another therapeutic group.

The consultant got us started. The program continues today under the direction of Dr. Cynthia Frazier, Director of Education and Clinical Programs at Morningside House. Additional educational programs have been given to all staff members on the Alzheimer's unit, and we are now expanding educational programs for all staff on all units.

Our philosophy of care embraces the primary care concept. All our primary caregivers have a specific primary assignment; thus, all residents have a permanently assigned primary caregiver. Establishing relationships is rarely easy; it may be even more difficult for residents with dementia. The primary care concept promotes not only relationships, but also continuity of care and accountability—all valuable components of a therapeutic environment.

Staff are vital to a therapeutic environment; they must be nurtured if they are going to be nurturing. In addition to education sessions, we conduct ventilating groups to allow the staff the opportunity to discharge some of the frustration they feel about caring for Alzheimer's patients.

The skilled nursing Alzheimer's unit is a success. Our turnover rate on the unit is minimal; there is a high degree of loyalty to the patients and to the unit; and staff members exhibit well-justified pride in the jobs they are doing.

Families

Families are intimately involved in the therapeutic environment. They are invited to participate in developing the plan of care. For example, they share with staff idiosyncracies about their resident that are crucial to helping us provide quality care and that could take ages for us to discover unaided. Families also participate in the care, where possible, and take part in a family support group. Including the family wherever possible engenders mutual trust and minimizes the potential for an adversarial relationship between staff and family. Family involvement promotes a team approach to care.

Physical Environment

Our physical surroundings are key to our sense of well-being. To assist us in creating a therapeutic physical environment, we engaged the services of Lorraine G. Hiatt, Ph.D., an environmental psychologist-gerontologist. Dr. Hiatt responded to our need by utilizing color and texture to help enable patients to know where they are and acoustical wall and floor coverings and carpet tiles to minimize environmental noise that exacerbates confusion. Each resident's room is designed to be uniquely recognizable in color and texture; we encourage families to bring a favorite small item such as a side table, picture, or afghan to personalize each room. We use "touch me" lamps that are turned on, made brighter, and turned off by the touch of a resident's hand.

Conclusion

A facility can create a therapeutic environment if that is its mission. It does not require extra space; it requires commitment. I believe one of the reasons our unit was so successful is that we shared our dream and commitment with staff and families, who responded by participating wholeheartedly in developing this project and in supporting the concept.

We have been so successful that our residents on this unit have been deemed by New York State to be low intensity in care. Unfortunately, since reimbursement is based on intensity of care, this environment has had a negative impact on our reimbursement. We use maximum resources to develop a resident who appears to require minimal care. It is a paradox. Nonetheless, the therapeutic environment is a major contribution to the quality of life for our residents, and that of course, in the long run, is what we are all about.

A Nationwide Survey of Special Units

Audrey S. Weiner

Report of Phase One of the Data Collection

In 1983, The Hebrew Home for the Aged at Riverdale (HHAR) made the decision to develop a third special care unit within its existing SNF bed complement. Unfortunately, at that time the literature provided little insight into the state of the art for special programs for the institutionalized Alzheimer's patient (Benedict 1983). Within our local community, we were able to identify only two special care units. We struggled to determine the optimal environment, staffing patterns and training, and models for a therapeutic milieu. Our frustration was mitigated only partially by our recognition that nationally *The Secretary's Task Force on Alzheimer's Disease* had identified as a priority for research to:

> "study the range of . . . institutional services relevant to Alzheimer's disease and related disorder patients in terms of their design, staffing, timing of use during the progression of the disorder, mix and coordination with other services and costs." (U.S. Department of Health and Human Services 1984).

Today, the literature does provide additional perspectives on this issue, including *Guide to Caring for the Mentally Impaired Elderly*, published by the American Association of Homes for the Aging (AAHA 1985). However, a recent survey of AAHA's membership indicated a significant interest in focusing on staff needs and on design and environmental concerns in order to develop programs for this special population (Webb 1985).

Through the support of The Brookdale Foundation, The Hebrew Home for the Aged at Riverdale has had the opportunity to identify and survey nationally institutions with special units and programs for residents with dementia. An overview of the special care unit responses for this population follows. Specifically, this report addresses articulated objectives, admission and discharge criteria, staffing patterns and training, daily recreational activities, and the integration of family supports.

This first phase of the study is based on information received, to date, from 27 facilities nationwide.

- Twenty completed facility survey forms.

- Five were interviewed on the telephone.

- Two were visited.

- Two provided written information.

- Twenty-two were nonprofit; five were proprietary.

Objectives of a Special or Designated Unit

Unfortunately, due to time constraints, the development of philosophy or objectives is often viewed as an intellectual luxury. In the development of special care units or programs, however, it is important that an operational framework, philosophy, or series of objectives be established.

Program objectives or goals articulated most frequently by those facilities surveyed include the following:

1. to provide a safe and secure environment which is supportive from both a nursing and a socialization perspective;

2. to reduce feelings of anxiety and confusion through both environmental and communication supports;

3. to rehabilitate or maintain the patient at an optimal level of physical and cognitive function;

4. to provide care to the patient in a holistic manner;

5. to recognize that these patients have come to facilities to

live, rather than merely to exist; and to provide experiences and activities that add to the quality of their lives;

6. to recognize that residents are autonomous human beings who can expect that their special needs and those of their families will be met with sensitivity and appropriateness;

7. to provide each resident with opportunities to succeed that serve to build his or her sense of self-esteem, dignity, and hope; and

8. to support the caretakers (staff, families, and significant others) through understanding, training, education, and the minimization of stress (AAHA 1985; Weissman 1984; Peppard 1984; Clark 1982; and Weiner 1985).

In addition, some facilities specifically indicate clinical goals including:

- the elimination of restraints
- the elimination of diapers and catheters for the incontinent patient
- the minimization of psychotropic drugs.

The decision to develop a special care unit goes well beyond its articulation and includes, at the outset, the development of such admission and discharge requirements as:

- determinations of age criteria
- behavior and functional criteria for admission and discharge
- priority for in-house residents.

Seventeen facilities indicated that patients were placed according to their level of cognitive/behavioral function. Of these, two facilities indicated that this was but one component of a more comprehensive system of patient placement based upon functional assessment. Within the remaining 15 facilities, special care units can be categorized as follows:

Number of Facilities		Type of Unit
9		short-term placement unit, from which a patient is discharged to traditional SNF when:
	5	• unresponsive to structured approach
	5	• in need of increased physical care
	3	• nonambulatory
	1	• extremely disruptive
3		multiple units with progressive intra-unit placement
3		long-term or permanent placement unit
15		

Admission to the Unit

Of the 15 units surveyed in depth, five identified their programs as serving individuals with mild to moderate dementia who were not part of a larger, progressive institutional system of placement. It should be noted that there was no relationship between this definition and the level of care (i.e., SNF or ICF).

The majority of facilities utilized a combination of functional and behavioral assessments. The four identifying diagnosis as a criterion noted that it was only a criterion for placement when linked to other behavioral and functional measures. Only four facilities reported use of validated assessment tools such as the Mental Status Quotient.

The Jewish Home for the Elderly of Fairfield County, Fairfield, Connecticut, links diagnosis, behavioral and functional criteria, and level of cognition as criteria for admission.

Jewish Home for the Elderly of Fairfield County Admission Criteria Bennett 2—Special Care Unit

1. The resident must fall within one of these three groups:
   a. needs direction to function in a familiar surrounding and can respond to instruction

    b. needs assistance to function and cannot respond to direction alone

    c. needs assistance to function and cannot communicate verbally in a meaningful fashion

2. Medical diagnosis of dementia

3. Mini-mental Status Score of 0 to 20

4. On the Geriatric Assessment Scale described below, the resident must score:
   a. a mean of 2.5 or less in all areas of the scale
   b. in the range of 3 to 6 in any category on the scale

5. Physician's approval

6. Family's consent

7. Persons with schizophrenia or a severe personality disorderwill not be eligible for the unit.

Here is the Geriatric Assessment Scale used to obtain scores for admission criterion number four above:

Jewish Home for the Elderly of Fairfield County Geriatric Assessment Scale

Please circle the most appropriate number in each category.

Eating and Nutrition

0   Self-care, weight steady
1   Needs prompting to eat, history of weight loss
2   Needs food cut up, wanders from table
3   Voraciously interested in sweets, steals food, marked weight gain, marked weight loss
4   Improper use of utensils, uses fingers, slight weight gain, eats inappropriate items, refuses to eat
5   Requires moderate to maximum assistance with eating
6   Tube fed, dysphagic, must be fed

Bowel and Bladder

0 Self-care
1 Asks to go, needs cues to locate toilet
2 Remindable, poor hygiene occasionally, forgets to flush
3 Regular supervision, requires assistance, occasionally incontinent of urine
4 Unpredictable, control by enema, occasional diapers, utilizes inappropriate areas for elimination
5 Frequent urinary and/or fecal incontinence
6 Fully incontinent, full-time diapers, full-time catheter for incontinence

Sleep

0 Sleeps through night, no interruptions, with or without medication
1 Wakens infrequently, returns to sleep without intervention
2 Wakens intermittently, may or may not require intervention
3 Wakens frequently, minimal intervention required
4 Wakens frequently, does not go back to sleep
5 Wanders regularly during sleeping time, calls out, has night and day reversed
6 More periods of sleep than wakefulness in a 24-hour period

Dressing

0 Dresses appropriately without instructions or help
1 Needs clothes set out, requires more directions and guidance
2 Inappropriate dress, misidentification of clothing
3 Won't change clothing, wears others' clothing
4 Will not leave clothing on, resists getting dressed
5 Requires moderate to maximum assistance for dressing
6 Must be completely dressed, unaware of need to dress

Grooming

0 Well groomed, attends to cleanliness, hair, teeth, clothing, toileting, shaving needs

1 Requires reminders to tend to daily hygiene and grooming tasks
2 Attends to some self-care grooming, but ignores others
3 Needs direction and assistance in grooming tasks
4 Resists hygiene routines: bathing, shaving, toileting
5 Requires moderate to maximum assistance in bathing, shaving, toileting
6 Unaware of need for grooming, food on face, hands, clothes

Sensory-Perceptual

0 Perceives environment accurately related to vision, hearing, taste, touch, and smell
1 Some difficulty distinguishing or identifying sensory input, e.g., poor vision or hard of hearing, etc.
2 Difficulty identifying human/nonhuman objects within environment
3 Body parts disorientation, misidentifies objects, difficulty with spatial concepts
4 Cannot distinguish or identify most visual or auditory input (can relate to touch, taste, or smell)
5 Agitated when sensory stimulation offered, tactile defensiveness, visual/auditory hallucinations
6 No apparent awareness or response when offered stimulation by touch, taste, or smell

Motor Coordination

0 Fully coordinated, good strength, range of motion
1 Responsive to commands, underactive, overactive
2 Occasionally requires assistance with mobility
3 Poorly coordinated, slow moving, stumbling
4 Involuntary movements, immobile, requires increased assistance and positioning
5 Wheelchair for safety, moderate to maximum physical assistance to ambulate
6 Immobile, unable to ambulate or initiate purposeful movement, contracted or spastic limbs, chin on chest

Cognitive

0   Bright, responsive, oriented, aware of surroundings
1   Forgetful, can be reminded or directed, can attend to activities
2   Impaired recent memory, confusion related to time and place, decreased attention span, easily distracted
3   Can be engaged sporadically and briefly, at times recognizes familiar environment and routine
4   Unable or unwilling to follow directions, cannot recognize familiar environment and routine
5   Impaired recent and remote memory, impaired body awareness
6   Disoriented to person, poor safety judgment and awareness

Memory-Familial

0   Recognizes and remembers all immediate family members
1   Recognizes and remembers all immediate family members other than grandchildren
2   Recognizes and remembers all family members except those by marriage
3   Recognizes and remembers siblings only
4   Recognizes and remembers family members intermittently
5   Recognizes but does not remember any family members by name
6   Does not recognize or remember any family members; speaks only of parents

Language-Conversation

0   Conversational
1   Repeats self, searches for synonyms, reticent conversation
2   Confabulates, white lies, mild vocabulary limitation, easily led in conversation
3   Loses thread of thought, noticeable vocabulary loss
4   Less aware of mistakes, poor syntax and sequence, perseveration, gives different meaning to words

5   Parrots words, incoherent, uncomprehending, severe vocabulary limitation
6   Totally nonverbal

Psychosocial

0   Cooperative, eager to participate in activities, takes initiative or can follow directions, selectively participates in activity according to interest and ability
1   Willingness to cooperate for short span of time, somewhat withdrawn, apathetic, but can be encouraged to participate
2   Sometimes reluctant to socialize or participate, prefers group, prefers one-to-one
3   Low frustration tolerance, cooperates only with identified person and routine, requires moderate encouragement
4   Demonstrates mood swings from acceptance to defiance, unwilling and/or unable to follow directions
5   Agitated and resistant when approached, paranoid system, delusional, unwillingness to socialize with others, provocative behavior, potentially harmful to self or others
6   Unable to socialize with peers, staff, or family, does not participate in any activities

The following shows The Hebrew Home for the Aged's criteria for admission to and transfer to the special units:

Criteria for Admission to Specialized SNF Units

To be admitted to this unit, patients will meet the following criteria:

I. *Cognitive*

Patient will have moderate to severe cognitive decline as indicated by one or more of the following:

* decreased knowledge of current and recent events—disorientation to time (day of week, season, etc.) or place

- exhibits deficit in memory of personal history (e.g., age, year married)
- concentration deficit elicited on serial subtractions (backward from 40 by 4: 40, 36, 32, and so on)
- inability to perform or follow through on complex tasks (such as dressing self) for functional reasons

And/or

II. *Behavioral* (observed and documented by staff)

- wandering into others' rooms, being disruptive or intrusive
- antisocial behavior—spitting, yelling, banging, fighting, undressing
- injurious behavior to self or others

And

III. *Physical*

- Physician's diagnosis of an organic mental disorder, i.e.,
  - a. primary degenerative dementia (DSM III 290.XX)
  - b. multi-infarct dementia (DSM III 290.4X)
  - c. Alzheimer's disease or SDAT, or
- A diagnosis of a major psychosis with behavior as described in II, i.e.,
  - a. schizophrenic disorder (DSM III 295.XX)
  - b. paranoid disorder (DSM III 297.XX)
  - c. bipolar disorder (with psychotic features) (DSM III 296.XX)

IV. *DSM-1 Measurement*

- Patient must have a DSM-1 score of at least 180. (Scores are generally well over 300).
- Total points for the mental status section will range from 85 to 210.

Note: Given the above cognitive/behavioral function, the patients considered for transfer will have a resultant need for greater or specialized assistance, support, and care.

Criteria for Transfer to Specialized SNF Units

I. *Diagnosis*

    a. Organic mental disorder (primary degenerative dementia, multi-infarct dementia, SDAT)

                                    _____   _____
                                       yes   no

    b. Major psychosis (schizophrenia, paranoia, bipolar disorder with psychotic features)

                                        _____   _____
                                       yes   no

If yes to either a or b, go on to II. If no to both a and b, then person does not meet criteria for transfer.

II. *Behavioral* (must be observed and documented):

	Nursing Notes	Social Worker Notes	Psychiatric Consultation
a. Wandering			
_____ yes _____ no			
b. Disruptive or intrusive			
_____ yes _____ no			

	Nursing Notes	Social Worker Notes	Psychiatric Consultation

c. Antisocial: Spitting,
yelling,
banging,
fighting,
undressing

—————   —————
yes   no

If yes to II, then person meets the criteria for transfer. If no to II, complete face-to-face interview to determine cognitives.

III. *Cognitive*

a. Disoriented to time

        ————— —————
        yes   no

b. Disoriented to place

        ————— —————
        yes   no

c. Deficit memory of personal history (age, year married)

        ————— —————
        yes   no

d. Serial subtractions—backwards from 40 by 4. (Write the numbers; document how far down the person went in the scale.)

        ————— —————
        yes   no

e. Documentation of inability to follow through on complex tasks for functional reasons (dressing, feeding, holding a cup)

        ————— —————
        yes   no

If yes to III or II, then person has met criteria for transfer. If no to both, then the person is not eligible.

f. The patient does _____ does not _____ meet the criteria for admission.

Environment

Approximately one-half of the facilities with special care units developed them through conversion from more traditional ICF or SNF units. There was a consensus about the importance of the environment for safety and security, orientation, organization and structure, and minimization of agitation and other behavior problems. The following lists the environmental modifications or supports within 22 facilities.

Environmental Modifications or Supports (22 Facilities)

	Number	Percent
1. Increased Security/Visual Access	18	82
• alarming, coding, securing exits	15	68
• modifying of nurse's station	3	14
• coding, securing, camouflaging elevators	3	14
• securing patio and garden areas	2	9
• using wide angle mirrors	2	9
• using television monitors	1	5
2. Increased Orientation	10	45
• reality orientation boards, large calendars, daily schedules	5	23
• color coding—corridors, furniture, etc.	5	23
• large letter/number/object room identification	4	18
• directional signs	1	5
3. Modification of Communal Space	8	36
• square footage increased	6	27
• garden or walkway created	3	14
• space modified to provide smaller areas for small group activities	1	5

	Number	Percent
4. Noise Control	7	32
• carpet tiles	5	23
• elimination of intercom or PA system	2	9

In addition:
- Two facilities utilize private rooms only.
- Two facilities are designed in a cluster of 6 to 8 patient rooms opening onto a communal day area.
- One facility indicates the addition of considerable texture for noise control and sensory stimulation.

As an example of environmental adaptations, in 1984, when The Hebrew Home was converting its traditional SNF unit to a special care unit, immediate modifications included placing alarms on exit doors, color coding corridors and doorways, installing wide angle mirrors, lowering the nurse's station, and increasing use of reality orientation boards and daily schedules. We accomplished the environmental changes within a few weeks at minimal cost and with minimal disruption. Later, at the suggestion of staff, we secured an adjacent garden area through the use of camouflaging planters. Pending recommendations include acoustical controls via the public address system.

Designation of special care units can become an issue. The overwhelming majority of facilities (71 percent) utilize their existing institutional nomenclature in referring to these units, for example, "E" Floor, Barnhard Unit.

- Two facilities call their special units "Life Enrichment Units."
- Two facilities refer to these floors as "Alzheimer's Unit" or "Alzheimer's Division."
- One facility had a staff contest to name its unit and now utilizes the acronym MIND which means maintaining independence in neuro-circulatory disorders (Fishkill Health Related Center, Beacon, New York).

Staffing

As indicated earlier, AAHA's membership identified staffing issues as serious concerns and priorities, especially given current regulatory constraints, the focus on cost containment, and the experience of other early research and demonstration projects wherein staffing ratios were impractical for the long-term care industry (Parker and Sommers 1983). In our survey, 14 skilled nursing facilities provided adequate information for staffing comparisons. Within these, facility size ranged from 120 to 784 beds, the number of dementia unit beds from 8 to 200. It should be noted that existing staff patterns were calculated and adjusted to a 40-bed SNF unit for ease of comparison. All facilities had at least one RN during the day and 13 had at least one RN during the evening.

Comparison of Special Care Unit Staffing at 14 SNF Facilities

	Nurses			Aides		
	Day	Evening RN + LPN	Night	Day	Evening	Night
Skilled Nursing	3.9	1.3	1.3	5.2	5.2	2.6
Facilities (SNF)	3.0	1.5	.75	4.5	3.0	3.0
	2.75	?	?	7.7	?	?
	2.6	1.9	1.3	5.7	4.3	2.6
	2.7	1.8	.9	5.4	4.5	2.7
	2.4	1.6	1.6	5.7	3.2	1.6
	2.4	2.4	1.6	6.4	4.8	4.8
	2.4	1.6	.8	6.6	3.3	1.6
	2.1	1.4	.7	4.2	4.0	3.0
	2.0	1.0	1.0	5.5	3.5	1.0
	2.0	1.0	1.0	6.5	4.5	2.5
	1.6	1.6	.8	7.0	5.2	3.5
	1.4	1.4	.3	5.2	5.3	1.3
	1.25	1.0	—	5.0	5.0	5.0
Health-Related Facilities (HRF) (Intermediate Care)	1.2	1.2	.9	3.5	3.5	2.7
Average by Category (SNF)	2.3	1.5	1.0	6.2	4.28	2.7
Median by Category (HRF)	2.4	1.5	.8	5.5	4.5	2.6

Indications of social work or recreational staff allocations were not consistent. Where these were included, however, there was a range from .4 full-time employees to 1, again based on that illustrative 40-bed unit example.

Several approaches to staffing merit note:

1. assigning activity workers to a 10 a.m. to 6 p.m. shift, which was more reflective of available program hours

2. locating social work and activity workers' offices on the special care units

3. using part-time feeders, assistants, or nurse's aides on the evening shift for feeding and assistance at bedtime

4. modifying traditional specific discipline or departmental responsibilities for tasks and activities.
   For example:

   • In three facilities, nurse's aides conduct reality orientation, remotivation, grooming, and activity programs. Two other facilities have plans to utilize this approach.
   • In three facilities, nurse's aide assignments are based on patient functional levels, allowing staff to conduct small group programs for persons at similar levels.

5. In four facilities, volunteers were sought from among staff, prior to the development of the special care unit, to work on this unit.

6. In five facilities (three nonprofit and two proprietary), there are coordinators for the special care unit whose time commitments range from half- to full-time with no relationship between either their existence, time allocation, or the number of designated special care beds. These individuals usually have the title of Clinical Coordinator with responsibility for program innovation, staff education, problem solving, and, within the proprietary facilities, program marketing. In one case, the coordinator is also responsible for actual programming on the unit.

Seventeen of the facilities completed information regarding the type and level of training, education, and staff supports provided within their special unit.

Staff Supports and Education (17 Facilities)

Response	Number	Percent
1. staff and team meetings (usually weekly) distinct from actual care planning sessions	11	65
2. training prior to the development of the unit	7	41
3. continued inservice	7	41
4. special training for new staff who will work on the special care unit	3	18
5. use of psychogeriatric hospital teams for clinical input, rounds, and education	3	18
6. team rounds	1	18

Facilities with regular staff and team meetings underscored their importance for ventilation and for discussion of specific clinical issues.

Initial training ranged from 12 to 40 hours and addressed the clinical course of dementia, its causes, expected changes in behavior, communication patterns, and useful strategies in relationships with patients and family members.

The experience of The Hebrew Home for the Aged at Riverdale underscores the importance of staff training throughout the facility. Beginning in 1982, an intensive educational effort had been developed distinct from the initiation of a special care unit. During the first year, all nurse's aides were trained in communication patterns and sensitivity toward the elderly, especially those with dementia. In the second year a multiple course series, conducted by the Hunter College Brookdale Center on Aging, addressed differential diagnosis, function related to dementia, communication, and other issues. In addition, staff found courses on psychotropic medications and on family relations most helpful. Regular staff meetings continue to be an essential part of the unit's operation.

Family Involvement

The survey indicated a clear understanding of the importance of support for family members.

Family Programs and Support (17 Facilities)

Program	Number	Percent
Family groups identified as:	14	82
• educational and emotional support groups	4	
• emotional support groups	4	
• educational groups	3	
• Alzheimer's disease support groups	3	
Family member programs that reflect total institutional approach (e.g., initial care planning conferences, preadmission orientation, annual care planning reviews)	6	35
Counseling	6	18

Activities

As we all know, institutional life, its demands and scheduling have a significant impact upon daily routines for our patients. Facility approaches to activities on dementia units vary from the highly structured, purposeful approach akin to The Burke Rehabilitation Model (Panella 1984) utilized, within five facilities, to a more flexible adaptation of institutional programs and weekly variety.

Simplistically, if we view a typical day in the context of meals and activities of daily living (ADL) schedules, we can identify activity time slots:

Daily Overview

Breakfast, morning care, toileting
- Two facilities utilize the breakfast time for announcements and orientation to the day's activity.
- On the average, two activity slots are scheduled for the morning.

Lunch, toileting, rest time
- one activity slot
- shift change
- a second activity slot

Dinner, toileting
- Six facilities indicated the existence of evening activities, often including music. Within two of these facilities, nursing staff conduct the activity.

The Fishkill Health Related Facility provides an excellent example of a structured approach to activities.

Structured Activities Approach—Fishkill HRF (ICF)
Selected Activities as Illustrative

Activity	What is Done	Purpose
Orientation 10:00	Introduce schedule of activities; current events; announcements; coffee	Give focus for the day; reinforce memory; promote group cohesiveness
Movement 10:45	Exercise; walking; dancing; music; bowling	Fitness; release tension; decrease wandering; stimulation
Lunch 11:30	Walk to dining room; conversation	Social stimulation; retention of social graces; continuity of life experience
Perception or Memory Recall Program 2:00	Puzzles; word games; bingo; discussion groups; music; cooking; crafts	Reinforce memory; promote concentration; creativity
Winddown 6:45	Review day's activities; relaxing techniques; lowering of lights; music for relaxing	Cues for slowing down

Facilities were also surveyed as to the type of activities conducted.

Activities Utilized Most Frequently on Special Units (in rank order)
(18 Facilities)

Program	Number	Percent
physical exercise (walks, adaptive sports, dance exercise, movement, wheelchair exercise)	15	83
music (singing, active/passive listening, "Mozart and wine")	10	56
reality orientation, remotivation	8	44
sensory stimulation, awareness, (conducted by Occupational Therapy Department)	8	44
cognitive stimulation (e.g., word games, communication, reminiscence)	5	28
crafts	5	28
bingo	3	17
grooming, basic skills classes	2	11
cooking	2	11
horticulture	2	11
pet therapy	2	11
ice cream and cocktail parties	2	11
sheltered workshop	1	6

This is similar to the successful ranking of activities noted by Mace (1984) in her survey of adult day care programs.

The activities most successful with demented clients in day care programs, in rank order, were:

- sing-alongs
- physical exercise
- walks
- reminiscence groups
- visits from children

- active games
- outings
- listening to music
- reality orientation
- visits from pets

Our survey overview makes clear that there is a core of accepted practices, including environmental adaptations, staff training and support, and family supports, that should be included in programmatic development, and that programs must fit within the context of each facility's own standards of practice, expertise, culture, and priorities.

References

American Association of Homes for the Aging. 1985. *Guide to caring for the mentally impaired elderly*. Washington, DC: AAHA.

Benedict, S. P. 1983. The decision to establish a closed psychiatric unit: Some ethical and administrative considerations. *The Journal of Long-term Care Administration: 22 - 26*.

Clark, E. T. 1982. A special nursing home unit for ambulatory demented patients. *Generations*: Fall.

Mace, N. 1984. Report of a survey of day care centers. *Pride Institute Journal of Long-term Health Care* 3(4):38 - 44.

Panella, J. R. and F. H. McDowell. 1984. Day care for dementia. The Burke Rehabilitation Center Auxiliary.

Parker, C. and C. Sommers. 1983. Reality orientation on a geropsychiatric unit. *Geriatric Nursing* 5:163 - 165.

Peppard, N. R. 1984. Giving holistic care: a special nursing home unit. *Generations:* Winter.

U.S. Department of Health and Human Services. 1984. *Alzheimer's disease: Report of the secretary's task force on Alzheimer's disease.*

Webb, M. 1985.Memorandum to AAHA Alzheimer's Disease Network.

Weiner, A. 1985. Developing a continuum of care for the individual with dementia and their family: Report of The Brookdale Planning Grant.

Weisman, S. 1984. A pilot program for the care of patients suffering from Alzheimer's disease and related dementias, presented at "National Perspectives on Alzheimer's Disease," Winston-Salem, NC.

Additional Reading

Devising Care Methods

Ackerman, J. O. 1985. Separated, not isolated—As basic as administrative backing and commitment. *Journal of Long-term Care Administration 13(3).*

Burnside, I. M. 1982. Care of the Alzheimer's patient in an institution. *Generations:* Fall.

_____. 1981. Unit Four in Nursing and the Aged, 2d ed. New York: McGraw-Hill.

Clark, T. A. 1982. A special nursing home unit for ambulatory demented patients. *Generations:* Fall.

The Fall 1982 issue of *Generations* is devoted to care of dementia patients from multidisciplinary perspectives; it includes a bibliography.

Hladik, P. Communicating with the Alzheimer's patient, from *Once I Have Had My Tea*. Available from the author at 419 Parsons Drive, Syracuse, NY 13219, for $3.00.

Mackey, A. M. 1983. OBS and nursing care. *Journal of Gerontological Nursing:* February.

McDowell, F. H., ed. 1980. *Managing the person with intellectual loss at home*. Burke Rehabilitation Center.

Shapira, J., R. Schlesinger, and J. L. Cummings. 1986. Distinguishing dementia. *American Journal of Nursing* 34(3).

Environment

Coutts, A. Elements and components of the environment planned for the Alzheimer's and dementia patient. Available from the author at Health Systems Specialist, 914 24th Street, Santa Monica, CA 90403.

Family Support

Information from the Alzheimer's Disease and Related Disorders Association (ADRDA), 360 North Michigan Avenue, Suite 601, Chicago, IL 60601.

To obtain "How to Organize a Self-help Group," mail request to National Self-help Clearing House, 33 West 42nd Street, New York, NY 10036.

Understanding Dementia and Differential Diagnoses

Cummings, J. L., and D. F. Benson. 1984. Dementia: *A clinical approach.* Woburn, MA: Butterworth Publishers.

Fisk, A. A. 1983. Management of Alzheimer's disease. *Postgraduate Medicine* 73(4).

Kennie, D. C., and J. T. Moore. 1980. Management of senile dementia. *American Family Practitioner:* December.

Special Units Or Programs for Individuals With Alzheimer's Disease

Nonprofit Facilities with Designated Special Units for Individuals with Dementia

Daughters of Israel Geriatric Center   201/731-5100
1155 Pleasant Valley Way
West Orange, NJ 07052

Ebenezer Caroline Center   612/879-2800
110 East 18th Street
Minneapolis, MN 55403

Green Hills Center   513/465-5065
6557 U.S. 68 South
West Liberty, OH 43357

Greenwood House   609/883-5391
Home for the Jewish Aged
53 Walter Street
Trenton, NJ 08628

Handmaker Jewish Geriatric Center   602/881-2323
2221 North Rosemont Boulevard
Tucson, AZ 85712

The Hebrew Home for the Aged at Riverdale   212/549-8700
5901 Palisade Avenue
Bronx, NY 10471

Hebrew Home of Greater Washington   301/881-0300
6121 Montrose Road
Rockville, MD 20852

The Indianapolis Jewish Home, Inc.   317/251-2261
(Hooverwood)
7001 Hoover Road
Indianapolis, IN 46260

Jewish Center for Aged   314/434-3330
13190 South Outer 40 Road
Chesterfield, MO 63017

Jewish Home for the Elderly   203/374-9461
   of Fairfield County
175 Jefferson Street
Fairfield, CT 06432

Marian Catholic Home   414/344-8100
3333 West Highland Boulevard
Milwaukee, WI 53208

Menorah Park Center for the Aging   216/831-6500
27100 Cedar Road
Beachwood, OH 44122

Morningside House   212/863-5800
1000 Pelham Parkway
Bronx, NY 10461

Philadelphia Geriatric Center   215/456-2900
5301 Old York Road
Philadelphia, PA 19141

St. John of God   213/731-0641
   Nursing Hospital and Residence
2035 West Adams Boulevard
Los Angles, CA 90018

Seven Acres-Jewish Home for the Aged   713/771-4111
6200 North Braeswood
Houston, TX 77674

Shalom Geriatric Center   816/333-7800
7801 Holmes Road
Kansas City, MO 64131

Wesley Homes, Inc.   404/728-6508
Budd Terrace
1833 Clifton Road, N.E.
Atlanta, GA 30029

Nonprofit Facilities Indicating Special Programs for Individuals with Dementia

Benedictine Nursing Center   503/845-6841
540 South Main Street
Mount Angel, OR 97362

Beth Abraham Hospital   212/920-5881
612 Allerton Avenue
Bronx, NY 10467

Hebrew Rehabilitation Center for Aged   617/325-8000
1200 Centre Street
Boston (Roslindale), MA 02131

Jewish Home for the Aging   818/881-4411
  of Greater Los Angeles
18855 Victory Boulevard
Los Angeles, CA 90048

Levindale Hebrew Geriatric   301/466-8700
  Center & Hospital
Belvedere & Greenspring Streets
Baltimore, MD 21215

Taylor Care Center   904/731-8230
6535 Chester Avenue
Jacksonville, FL 32217

Margaret Tietz Center for Nursing Care   718/523-6400
164-11 Chapin Parkway
Jamaica, NY 11432

**Proprietary Facilities with Special Units
for Dementia Patients**

Courtland Gardens Health Center   203/359-2000
59 Courtland Avenue
Stamford, CT 06902

Fairfield Manor Health Care Center   203/853-0010
23 Prospect Avenue
Norwalk, CT 06850

Fishkill Health Related Center, Inc.   914/831-8704
Route 9-D and Dogwood Lane
Beacon, NY 12508

Hillhaven Corporation has 12 to 15 active special units scattered about the country, including Newton-Wesley, Kansas City, Phoenix, Denver, Portland, and San Francisco.

List of self-identifying facilities was compiled by The Hebrew Home for the Aged at Riverdale.

Chapter 6

Care for the Caregivers

The Burdens of Caregivers

Steven H. Zarit

The purpose of this section is to provide an overview of the problems faced by caregivers and of strategies for alleviating the stress or burden that they experience.

By burden I mean the caregiver's subjective sense that caregiving activities are burdensome to his or her physical health, emotional health, or social life. Burden is a subjective concept; that is, it is not my judgment that a particular caregiver or family is caring for a patient in ways that are detrimental. It is the caregiver's own feeling that the caregiving is having detrimental effects.

Often I might make the assessment that what a family does for an Alzheimer's patient is having a negative impact on the lives of its members, but they say, "No, we can do it; we are able to manage; things are going okay." In other instances, I might make the assessment that the caregiver ought to be able to care for the individual, but the caregiver says, "No, it is overwhelming, and I can't manage any more." The caregiver's burden is subjective.

Most of the studies of caregiver burden, including my own, have been done on samples of caregivers who are caring for an individual who is still in the community. Very little work has focused on caregivers of institutionalized Alzheimer's or other dementia patients.

However, both from the limited research available and from case examples, it is apparent that the caregiver's burden does not stop at the door of the institution. Several studies suggest that the caregiver's burden is not alleviated by institutional placement; rather, the sources of burden shift. The caregivers may not be providing round-the-clock care any more, but they continue to visit. They may be traveling long distances which may be another source of stress for elderly caregivers. They are also interacting with the staff to try to ensure certain kinds of care. There is the additional financial burden that institutional care places on them.

In one of our recent studies—a longitudinal study following caregivers who were all spouses—contrary to expectations, we found that wives who placed their relatives in institutions were reporting that they were more socially isolated after placement and that their need for support and interaction with other people had actually increased after the placement.

Health professionals may do a disservice to families when they advise them that the way to ease their burden is to place their relative in a facility. That solution may create inappropriate expectations and serve only to shift the emphasis of their burden.

The caregivers' ongoing emotional burden—guilt, anger, depression, and fear—will complicate care in any setting, including a long-term care setting. Sometimes their emotional stress results in staff and family conflicts or in continuing conflicts within the family over what is the right thing to do with the Alzheimer's patient.

Sources of Burden

Health professionals tend to make the assumption that the disease causes the burden. Since doctors cannot change the course of Alzheimer's disease to any great extent, we assume we cannot do anything about the caregiver's burden.

But there are mediating factors that determine whether caregivers experience more or less burden. In our research, we see caregivers assisting patients with the most severe impairments who report little or no burden. Yet we see other caregivers caring for patients with very mild deficits who report severe burden. The reason for the discrepancies is that there are factors aside from the patient's disability that account for how much burden the family, and particularly the primary caregiver, experiences.

An important factor in determining how much burden the family will experience is its response to the care demands caused by the patient's illness: disruptive behavior, need for assistance with the activities of daily living, and so on. Some caregivers manage these problems well, some manage them poorly; some understand why the patient behaves the way he or she does, others do not.

Another factor is how much social support caregivers have; social support can range from receiving active assistance to simply having an understanding person with whom to talk.

A third important factor is the quality of the prior family relationship. Families come in all shapes and sizes. There is probably nothing more varied in society than family structure and the way that family members interact with each other. Each family situation is unique; therefore, first we must learn about the family's structure and its psychological makeup. We begin by asking: Who is the caregiver? What is that caregiver's relationship to the patient? It makes a difference, for example, whether the caregiver is a spouse or a child. Spouses are much more strongly invested in the care of patients than are their children, but it can be easier for children than for spouses to use services including long-term care. It is also important to consider whether the spouse is a husband or a wife. Our research has shown that wives seem to have a more difficult time as caregivers than do husbands. They experience much greater emotional distress and are therefore more difficult to work with because their resources are stretched thinner from the outset.

The better the quality of the past relationship, the less burdened the caregiver will be, regardless of whether the caregiver is husband, wife, son, or daughter.

The family's psychological makeup is a final important factor. Was this a close family or a distant one? Was it harmonious or marked by conflict? What was the role of the patient in the family? The role he or she played may be crucial for understanding the family's response.

If the patient was the family's organizer, the person who got things to happen, or the person to whom everyone turned for emotional support, then the patient's illness can be particularly disruptive. The family is likely to have more trouble mobilizing to provide support to the patient and the primary caregiver.

Similarly, the accustomed role as the caregiver is important to understand. If the caregiver is the central person in the family, people will rally around that individual. If the caregiver is seen as weak or ineffectual or as having problems of his or her own, then the family may not rally around to provide assistance.

Strategies for Relieving Stress

The manner in which caregivers respond to symptoms—both what caregivers understand about the patient's disease behavior and the particular coping responses they use for dealing with problem behavior—determines whether their stress is aggravated or eased.

In our research, we found that understanding the patient's problem is crucial and that caregivers do better when they get their questions answered. Sometimes doctors spend time answering questions; sometimes they do not. At times, when caregivers first hear the answers, they are under too much stress to process the information well. We find it important to spend some time providing information about what the disease is; what causes it, or at least what we know about what might cause it; what possible treatments are; what the best care for the patient might be; and so on. We also spend a lot of time providing information about effects of the disease on patients' behavior. Caregivers experience needless stress because they misinterpret why patients do what they do.

There are many misinterpretations. When a patient asks the same question over and over again, the family sometimes assumes the patient is trying to annoy them, that the patient could really control the behavior, or that he or she is lazy. "He is not remembering because he is not trying."

In everyday circumstances, those could be appropriate interpretations, but when an individual suffers global brain damage as in the case of Alzheimer's disease or the other dementias, the patient cannot remember asking the question before, even if it was only two minutes earlier. We try to help families understand the patient's disability.

Again, when a relative makes a false accusation—"You are stealing things."—it is very upsetting to families. It contradicts their understanding of what really happened, and they get upset. The family concludes that the patient is crazy or malicious, rather than understanding that the reason patients make accusations is that they cannot remember where they put the lost item.

Pointing out the mistakes to the patients does not help; they become upset because their memory loss creates in them a strong sense of insecurity. They cannot find things or remember what they have done with them. To say that an object has been stolen is a normal defensive response.

The approach we take with families is to encourage them first to see the patient's problems as part of a disease. Then, if reasoning with the patient is not working, we encourage them to respond by empathizing, that is, trying to understand the feelings behind the patient's statement or behavior. Thus, instead of arguing over the facts regarding whether or not an item was stolen, the family might say, "It must be upsetting; I know you are upset. It must be hard not to be able to find things." Often that response will have a calming effect when reasoning does not.

To cite an example, a man who was the caregiver got into an argument with his wife, who had dementia. She was concerned about a bank account that they had closed out ten years earlier. He had always taken care of the money in their relationship, and he felt she was criticizing the way he managed the money. He would say, "Look, we closed it out," and she would say, "I want to go to the bank." The more he reasoned with her, the more angry she became. The more angry she became the more upset he became, because he felt that she was questioning his competency. The solution in that situation was, first, to sit down with him and ask him why she might be doing this and what she might be feeling.

asking because she could not remember. Even though he
...ys been responsible for money matters, she had been involved and now felt insecure since she could no longer keep track of money.

We taught him to respond to her insecurity rather than to what she was saying. The next time she brought it up, he said, "I am taking care of everything; we have plenty of money." That reassured her, and she stopped asking the question.

She really had been asking, "Do we have enough money? Are we secure?" Not, "Can I see this bank account?"

This example relates to other problems with words demonstrated by Alzheimer's patients. They use words in inappropriate or strange ways, and caregivers have trouble understanding. The patients are either misusing words or misremembering the words they want and substituting others. A mild aphasia or word-finding problem is found in most early cases of Alzheimer's disease, and this problem gradually worsens.

Patients also lose the ability to follow multiple commands, for example, "Go in the next room and bring me the newspaper." Because of their memory loss, they might only be able to do the first thing. They get into the next room but cannot remember what the second part of the command is. The problem is compounded with a command like, "Go get dressed." They go into the bedroom and forget the rest. Then the caregiver and the patient get into a fight over dressing.

We have found that giving patients one command at a time is very helpful. A caregiver said, "Go ahead and sit down," to her husband who would stand up and pace during periods of agitation. In response he would go ahead by taking a couple of steps forward, and then he would stop. He would not sit because he had forgotten the second part of the command. She then realized that she had to make two statements in order for her husband to follow her direction. Breaking commands into the smallest possible steps can help when patients are unable to remember a complex command.

Alzheimer's patients also have perceptual problems. They will look at an object, perhaps even be able to name it but will not know its function. For example, problems related to bathing may occur because patients no longer know what the bathtub is used for; they become frightened. Using the word to explain its function does not help because they may not understand the meaning of the word.

One of the most dramatic examples of the impairment in Alzheimer's disease is revealed when patients take a naming test. Shown common, familiar objects such as bathtubs, chairs, and tables, they can name them but cannot explain their use.

When naming and function problems start developing and ordinary objects become frightening to the patient, it is helpful to think about why the patient might be frightened. If the caregiver is able to understand what the patient is going through, he or she is better able to control problem behaviors. If the patient gets upset and the caregiver responds by getting equally upset, the problem escalates. A caregiver who is able to respond empathetically can often calm the patient.

Six Steps for Problem Solving

Another important factor in relieving caregiver burden is problem solving. Problem solving is a strategy for identifying ways to better control problem behavior.

To modify problem behavior, we go through a series of steps in problem solving. Let me use as an example a patient who is not sleeping at night, a problem that causes stress at home or in institutions.

First, we identify the problem clearly: how often is it occurring and in what circumstances? In identifying the problem, we would track how often the patient is getting up at night, what the patient is doing during the day, and whatever other antecedents are causing the problem. A common cause of not sleeping at night is napping during the day.

Next, we brainstorm with the caregivers to generate solutions. We ask them to think of anything that comes to mind and to free associate in order to devise possible solutions. As a third step, we encourage them to select a solution from the discussion of possible strategies. Step four is to rehearse the solution with them to identify any reasons that might prevent it from working.

Fifth, we encourage them to carry out the plan, and sixth, we evaluate the outcome. If the plan is not successful, we look at possible reasons why it is not working and then start the process over.

This approach for managing behaviors has been applied to problems such as poor sleeping, incontinence, repetitious questioning, agitation, and restlessness. Often, a plan and an intervention can be developed to control those behaviors. Now that this approach has been successful in home settings, we are applying it in a special Alzheimer's unit. The staff is finding it successful for dealing with a variety of problems. Patients who were incontinent, for example, have been placed on schedules to reestablish their toileting habits. By setting schedules so that intervals are shorter than the time in which they wet or soiled themselves, it is now possible to keep them clean and dry. This approach has been successful with patients who had been incontinent for over one year on a regular nursing unit.

Support for Caregivers

Caregivers have continuing needs for emotional or physical support. The need for emotional support is met by providing a nonjudgmental listener, someone to whom the caregiver can talk.

In addition, caregivers may need certain kinds of assistance. They may be frail and need physical help; they may need help with transportation or with household tasks. A caregiver may never have managed the family finances and so may need financial counseling or assistance.

Support is often delivered through support groups, which work extremely well for a number of reasons. Not only do they provide the emotional support that caregivers need, but they provide it in a special way that professionals cannot because the support comes from other people going through the same experience.

Our research shows that support groups work better if they are organized around the caregiver's relationships: all spouses or all children. Mixing spouses and children is less effective. At times, mixing everyone together can be useful, but over the long term, groups organized according to the caregivers' relationship are better.

Mixing spouses, both husbands and wives, works nicely; they learn from each other's strengths and weaknesses. For example, one of our early support groups contained wives who were clearly stressed and had a great deal of trouble caring for their husbands at home. Whenever the group leaders brought up the options of getting someone in to help or of taking their husbands out to a day care program, the wives would say, "No, I should be able to do it. I should be able to do everything myself."

The husbands in the group, meanwhile, were experiencing some of the same problems, but they had received outside help. They reported to the group about the difference it made for them. The wives looked around at each other and said, "If they can do it, we can do it, too," so they went out and got help. That is the kind of learning that can occur in a support group.

Groups also need a skilled leader. A group can have a powerful effect on individuals, an effect that is not always positive. Groups can ignore or ostracize someone, they can scapegoat an individual in the group, or they can have other harmful effects.

A well-trained leader will maintain a therapeutic atmosphere, will head off these problems as they develop, and will redirect the group's interactions in a more positive way. To cite an example, we had one ongoing support group with strong cohesiveness; the group members, all spouses, were very close to each other. In one session, a relatively new member asked, "What about dating other people? What do you think about that?" That was a sensitive, even an explosive, topic. The group ignored the question. No one answered; instead, they started talking about something else. But the leader stopped them and said, "Wait a minute, what did he say?" The group started laughing at how all of them had heard him, but all had chosen to ignore his question. They brought this man back into the discussion, and for the rest of the session they had an animated discussion about dating. If the leader had not intervened, this new member would have felt ostracized, as though he were wrong to bring up the subject. By returning to the question, the leader had established that any topic related to the caregiving experience was fair game for the group to discuss. The discussion turned out to be helpful to all of them, not just to the man who brought it up.

It is important to recognize, however, that some individuals do not benefit from support groups. Some caregivers drop out of groups. Wives who are under a lot of stress tend to drop out before they form allegiances with group members or with the leader.

Our own studies show that about one-third of the caregivers who go into support groups actually show increased burden as a result of participation. Groups are not a universal cure-all.

Our findings suggest that, on average, caregivers receiving individual counseling find more benefit in that than in support groups; they get more insight into the problem and feel more support. They value the relationship with the counselor more.

Now, the differences between support groups and counseling are not large; groups work better for some people, individual counseling for others. Some people need more than a support group offers. For example, I prefer to work individually with someone under a great deal of stress.

Some people may not do well in a support group because of their personalities. If in an interview I have trouble getting a person to stop talking, that person may be difficult to keep from dominating discussion in a group. An individual with a personality disorder, very self-centered or prone to go off on tangents, can put too much stress on other members of a group. It is important to have other options available, including individual counseling.

The central question in adapting these approaches for long-term care facilities is: what role will the family have in the overall care plan? Families want varying degrees of involvement and have varying degrees of ability to help.

In an Alzheimer's unit in the Los Angeles area, we have been studying the effects of the care methods on families as well as patients. Families are permitted on the unit from ten o'clock in the morning until eight o' clock at night. The families are encouraged to be there. They can get meals there and under certain circumstances may stay overnight; so they feel involved with the program. That is not always a positive thing for the staff. Some families are helpful; others are difficult.

A key question concerns how to help families become more effective caregivers for the institutionalized dementia patient. One strategy involves including the caregiver in the treatment plan. We often assume incorrectly that families know why facilities do the things they do with patients. Taking the time to inform families of the rationale behind care methods is vital. For instance, if on a unit the staff were trying a problem-solving approach to manage certain behaviors, it would be important to make the caregivers an adjunct to that approach. Another strategy that helps the family feel a part of the team and the treatment plan is to demonstrate some rehabilitation and progress.

It is also important to communicate promptly to the family about both good and bad things. Of course, it is easy to communicate about the good things; it is harder to communicate sad news. Communication should come from someone with appropriate status. All too often the aides, rather than the nurse or the physician, communicate with the family. A third important strategy is to have places for patients and family to socialize together.

Another factor is balance: to encourage the family's involvement but not overwhelm them or the patient by scheduling too many activities. We like to keep patients active, but if the families are going to be there, quiet breaks are necessary to allow the family time to interact with the patient.

Finally, a homelike atmosphere is a key to success in Alzheimer's units. Since the facility is not providing medical care, there is no need for a hospital atmosphere. The amount of medical care on a typical Alzheimer's unit is confined to a few minutes each day. The more homelike the atmosphere, the more the families will be encouraged to visit and interact, and the more they will interact in normal ways.

This overview has considered sources of the caregiver's burden and strategies for dealing with that burden, both at home and in special Alzheimer's or dementia units in long-term care facilities.

Support Services For Families

Barbara J. Esposito

Today, with the rapidly growing aged population and the prevalence of intergenerational families, the need to work with the elderly and their families as integral parts of a family system is of utmost importance. When one member of a family system has Alzheimer's disease, the urgency is even greater. It should be an axiom in human services that an aged client is considered as a member of a larger family system.

Despite the myth that the elderly are dumped into nursing homes, statistics reveal that the vast majority are not in institutions, that only 5 percent are in long-term care facilities. We cannot, however, falsely assume that those 5 percent in institutions have been abandoned by families or are without families, though some may be. It has been my experience that the devastation of some disease process has necessitated placement in a long-term care facility as the only reasonable, safe, and humane care to offer a family member.

Normal developmental aging itself can be a source of anxiety and stress to certain family units. Alzheimer's disease and eventual institutionalization are a crisis for the individual, but they also become a crisis for the significant others in the family. Most of the impact is on the adult children of Alzheimer's patients. The family support services at The Jewish Home for the Elderly are offered primarily to adult children of the residents on our unit, where the mean age of the resident is 86.

Families operate as emotional units; what affects one member of the family must have some impact on all others. A diagnosis of Alzheimer's disease and subsequent admission to a long-term care facility (LTCF) will certainly affect not only the afflicted individual but others in the family. It is not only the physical separation of the individual who has gone to reside in a long-term care facility that can create havoc in family members, it is also the forced resurgence of the lifelong process of emotional separation that comes into play at this time. Individuals throughout their adult lifetimes undergo the emotional process of breaking dependent ties with parents and establishing independence. This process is an ambivalent one and still can be unresolved at the time a parent enters a long-term care facility. Even if this process has been worked through, placement can evoke strong feelings in adult children. It is, then, our responsibility in long-term care to be cognizant of these issues and work with the entire family as well as the individual client.

For families who care for a loved one with Alzheimer's disease at home and who fight to keep their sanity as they cope with the inherent difficulties of such care, admission of a demented family member to a long-term care facility is all too often a needed respite. It is most often the best and only choice for families. However, this respite often takes the form of a permanent placement and can have a high emotional cost to family members. Should this occur in a family where cultural and ethnic beliefs dictate that children should care for aged parents, emotional upheaval is intensified.

Someone once remarked to me that family members of the residents on our special care unit for Alzheimer's patients must not require a great deal of support. "After all," this person stated, "they are not primary caregivers and are no longer dealing with the anxieties of caring for this person at home." While it is true that these family members are not primary caregivers and that the issues they must cope with are different from primary family caregivers, they still require a great deal of support. They can suffer a great deal of psychic pain and as much anguish as family members providing care at home. Often the admission to long-term care comes after an extended period of being a primary caregiver, and the person's coping repertoire is already taxed.

When a family member is placed in a nursing home for Alzheimer's patients, the caregiver's respite is permanent. Whether stated or unstated, accepted or denied, the reality of the situation is that the impaired family member will spend the rest of his or her life in the facility and will ultimately die there. Families are unique, and how the family copes with this situation and with the subsequent progression of the disease process depends on a myriad of factors. Factors to be aware of include:

- the quality of the relationship between the client and other family members
- the family's cultural and ethnic background
- the family's prior coping styles
- prior contacts, if any, with the long-term care facility
- prior support and education, if any, regarding Alzheimer's disease
- the attitude of the nursing home staff as perceived by the family.

It should be noted that some of these phenomena are operational on admission to a long-term care facility even when a condition other than dementia exists. Families may experience difficulty also if a family member, who is in a long-term care facility due to a medical condition, starts to exhibit signs of dementia. They may fault the institution for the relative's decline and deny the presence of an irreversible dementia of unknown etiology. Also, families may experience difficulty when a relative must be transferred from an intermediate level of care to skilled care.

When a resident is transferred to our special care unit, a skilled nursing unit, families usually react in one of two ways. To some, the *special care unit* conjures up thoughts of special treatment, perhaps fantasies of the process of Alzheimer's being stopped. To still other families, to consent to a transfer to the special care unit means leaving intermediate care; it means that the relative has declined and is in need of even greater care. Clearly, the family needs support and education at this time.

Admission to a nursing home and the diagnosis of Alzheimer's disease can be a crisis for many families. Often unresolved family difficulties can resurface during such a crisis and further disrupt this difficult time. For example, unresolved sibling rivalry can resurface, with adult siblings at odds over who shall care for a parent and how. Formerly ambivalent feelings between parent and adult child can emerge and make the situation more traumatic.

In my work with families, I have observed both positive and negative coping styles in confronting both nursing home placement and admission to the Alzheimer's care unit. For learning purposes, the phases of these coping mechanisms are displayed in Figure 1.

As helping persons in long-term care, we strive to help families to deal in positive ways with the impact of a disease such as Alzheimer's and with institutionalization, yet remain aware in our own minds of the conflictual messages society often sends to adult children: be responsible for your aged parent, but at the same time be mature and independent, be separate, cut the proverbial apron strings. Families can often resolve the normal developmental stage of aging and illness in a member, but frequently will need help from a professional. We need to know what to look for and when to intervene, and we need a model to follow.

As coordinator of an inpatient unit, I come in contact with family members of 30 residents as well as families of residents elsewhere in the home. The fact that they are not primary caregivers does not negate the fact that these families need support. It is often precisely because families are not the primary caregivers that they need support.

Families are depending now on others to care for their loved ones. For some this is a true relief and results in a feeling of security. For others, the loss of control, the dependence on long-term care staff, generates a great deal of anxiety. For example, some families speak of being at the mercy of the staff. That loss of control precipitates anxiety. Still others have difficulty observing people outside the family giving quality care to mother or father in a way that they were not able to do. It is the continuing presence of a progressive disease, one unknown in terms of cause and cure, that admission to a long-term care facility forces families to confront.

For adult offspring, often the diagnosis of Alzheimer's and admission to a nursing home occurs simultaneously with what is described by Blenker (1965) as "filial crisis." Filial crisis is that time when adult children can look no longer to parents to be rocks of support but instead must themselves start to support the parent. Filial maturity is needed; parents need to be able to depend on their children for help. If this normal stage in adult development has not been resolved, further upheaval upsets the delicate balance of the family confronting dementia and placement of one of its members.

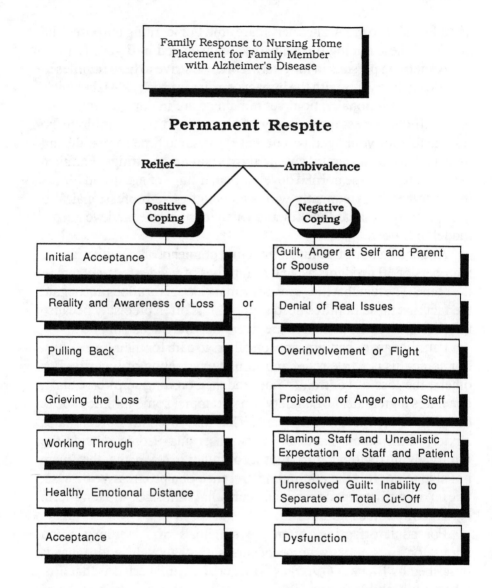

Permanent Respite

Figure 1. May Proceed Through the Phases Again as Additional Functional Losses Appear.

Let me share four case reports with you to illustrate some of the coping mechanisms and phases families experience in the long-term care setting. Some families move through this upheaval positively, falling back on former effective coping patterns of handling stress; others react using less effective means.

Case I. Eighty-five-year-old Mrs. P. had cardiac problems and Alzheimer's disease. In 1982, when she was still quite alert, she initiated her own placement at The Jewish Home for the Elderly and was satisfied with the facility. Mrs. P. had three daughters of whom one, Mary, was the primary contact. The resident's two other daughters lived out of state and visited infrequently. Mrs. P. was initially admitted to the rest home level of care, but as her dementia progressed, she was transferred to skilled care on the special unit.

Mrs. P's daughter related to staff her initial misgivings about seeing her mother enter a nursing home but stated that her mother's obvious satisfaction with the home had eased her concerns. The daughter was informed about the special care unit and saw it as a viable place for her mother to go when she could no longer function in the rest home. Mrs. P. eventually became very disoriented but pleasantly confused, and more and more apraxic and aphasic once on the special care unit. These new functional losses upset this daughter greatly, but she would seek staff out to talk and accepted these declines as part of her mother's illness.

This daughter began to volunteer on our unit, leading a weekly sing-along. The staff believed that she was able to gain support in this way and work through her feelings of sadness over her mother's changing condition. She could still reach both her mother and her mother's coresidents via music. This daughter would visit once or twice weekly.

Mrs. P. developed pneumonia over the course of a few months and died. Her daughter was able to cry for her mother, but she told the staff that she had begun letting go a little at a time and felt at peace because she had seen the high quality of life her mother had up to the end. At a three-month contact with her daughter, she stated: "I felt at peace when mother passed. I feel my volunteering helped. My sisters unfortunately have had a more difficult time."

Our staff encourages families to volunteer on our unit, if they are so inclined. It promotes a partnership between family and staff and can be a great means of helping families cope. Mrs. P's daughter obviously had the ability to handle this situation effectively, but this is not to say that she did not feel a great loss over her mother's decline and death.

I would like to interject at this point that despite mixed feelings on the part of some families towards a special unit for dementia, over time many of these families do accept the reality of their relatives' illness with greater ease than do families with demented relatives elsewhere in the facility. Relatives of those on the special care unit feel that something extra is being done for their family member and entertain the hope that special care will retard the functional decline. In addition, the expanded support services on the special care unit for the families themselves have a positive effect.

Case II illustrates a family member's initial acceptance of placement, then denial of the real issues of continuing cognitive loss in a family member, and finally difficulty accepting changes in the resident.

Mr. and Mrs. A. are a married couple on our unit, both diagnosed with Alzheimer's disease. They have an only son, B. The son will tell you that his mother does have Alzheimer's disease and talks openly about the progression of her dementia. The son will then say that his father does not have Alzheimer's disease; he just has normal memory problems due to his age. One only has to watch son and parents visit to see this family's love and warmth. The son's acceptance of his mother's dementia is evident, as is his overwhelming respect and identification with his father. This son can be called a model family member, one who had always been supportive of the staff, helpful and pleasant.

Mr. A., 92 years old and very active, began to decline, however, becoming very disoriented and anxious. His son was quite upset with the change and insisted that the doctor give his father a complete physical, stop certain medications, and visit more frequently. Simultaneously, this son demanded that the staff start challenging his father with higher functioning tasks to stimulate him. The son began to visit daily, started taking video movies of his parents and called the staff frequently from home. We see in this case sudden overinvolvement based on denial of the real issues—that a 92-year-old person with Alzheimer's disease does forget and does tire by 7:30 p.m.—and then unrealistic expectations of both staff and patient. We see a son in filial crisis. He was not ready to see his father dependent, telling himself that his father was in a nursing home only to keep his mother company. This is a son who must be frightened beyond belief, having not one but both parents with Alzheimer's disease.

Immediate intervention in a case like this is important. One-to-one counseling meetings were initiated and the son started attending a monthly support group offered to all family members of residents on our unit. He is beginning to accept his father's dementia, but only with great difficulty.

Case III. Mrs. Y's daughter visited daily. She was anxious and had been opposed to her mother's transfer to our unit. She pushed to keep her mother on the rest home level of care, despite the fact that her mother needed more supervision. A crisis ensued between the mother and her roommate, and there was no other choice but to send this resident from intermediate care to our unit. Once her mother was transferred, the daughter became hypervigilant, visiting at long intervals and watching staff closely, yet very concerned and cooperative. This daughter was eager to attend a support group and quite verbal in the group about how difficult both the diagnosis of Alzheimer's disease and admission to the home had been for her to handle. Her mother was doing well on the unit, prior paranoia and abusiveness all but dissipated, and the daughter's anxiety quelled. She has returned to work full time, visits weekly, and continues in the support group where she is working through this phase in her family's life cycle and is able to be supportive of other families, helping them to develop realistic expectations.

We may not need to help all families formally, although we need to be astute at observing the warning signals that tell us families need our intervention; we must anticipate this need. Some families unfortunately resist our efforts, as this last case illustrates.

Case IV. We have all worked with problem families. Mrs. I's daughter is that kind of family member that staff try to avoid; she is difficult even for the most understanding worker. Our staff continues to reach out to her, despite her resistance to accept help. This daughter wanted her mother on our unit, yet is never satisfied with any of the care or help rendered. Her mother is a very combative woman and the staff feel that their very best efforts at care are not good enough. This daughter frequently berates staff, her own mother, and other residents on the unit as well. Constant limit-setting is needed with this family member. This daughter challenges her mother, usually agitating her more. Instead of having a staff member distract her mother who cannot anticipate future visits, this daughter elicits her mother's cries of, "Don't go! Take me home!" because her own need to still be loved by mother takes precedence over the mother's distress.

On a few rare occasions, this daughter has wept and talked of her guilt and fear, but only infrequently does she uncover and confront her pain. She refuses to attend support groups and cancels one-to-one meetings. Other families have reached out to her, but to no avail. Clearly, this daughter is dysfunctional in this situation. We can continue to reach out to her, but we are aware that prior difficulties in the family and poor coping mechanisms in other life situations are probably operational here.

A Model for Support Services

Our interdisciplinary team has identified and focuses on three key areas in meeting the needs of families. Our goals in working with families are to inform, educate, and support the family. All three areas are equally important in reaching out to families and helping them confront and accept ongoing decline in their relatives.

Keeping families informed about the status of their loved one and about our overall program is probably one of our most important functions. The staff does not wait for families to call for updates on condition. If there are any changes in status, medication, or activity level, a call goes out to the family. We try to leave no surprises for family members when they arrive for visits; this proves very helpful.

Furthermore, meetings are often arranged between team members and families to clarify uncertainties and to work on a mutual plan of care.

A family information board provides information to families about resident activities and the overall program, as well as educational material on Alzheimer's disease. This board is located right on our unit where families visit.

Families often have questions about the diagnosis of dementia. Large group meetings, where families can hear speakers, view films, and ask questions, are aimed at meeting our goal of educating families. The unknown can generate anxiety; by educating and informing families, we alleviate fear of the unknown and convey our accessibility to the families, hopefully engendering trust.

Our goal in working with families is to make all aware—staff and families—of the mutual responsibility that is involved in the care of the resident. Staff, then, must also be educated to understand what the needs and concerns of families are. Staff need a supportive environment. They are now the primary caregivers; in addition, they must interact with families. If the staff feel supported, they can respond therapeutically to families, even difficult families who project their anger onto the staff.

Our ultimate goal in working with families of residents in long-term care is to provide the support they need as their relatives succumb to a progressive dementia. Education, information, and accessibility of staff help, and on our unit, a monthly support group has proved to be beneficial.

Family members were in such need of a support group, as evidenced by frequent calls, unrealistic expectations of residents and staff, and other issues brought out in earlier case presentations. Several families openly asked for a support group. At the first meeting, family members were not reticent; in fact, there was such a need to talk about the painful experience they were enduring that most group members verbalized at great length. Therapeutically, it is best for group members not to verbalize too much at the first group, lest they feel that they have exposed too much and not return. Some members remarked after the first group that perhaps once a month was too frequent for meetings, yet all have returned each month. At subsequent group sessions, members were more hesitant and focused on intellectual issues, such as diagnosis, cause, and cure, yet this is an important group process. The catharsis at the first group, with families relating about all they did to keep the parent at home for as long as possible, was necessary and showed that these family members need support by peer family members who share the same feelings.

The group is one of the best ways to offer families support. One only has to hear a relative remark to another resident's relative, "I thought I was the only one who felt that way," to know that the group is the modality of choice.

Other issues that are common to long-term care facility groups for Alzheimer's family members are:

- fear and concern about Alzheimer's being a hereditary disease

- reality of the group member's own aging

- guilt over long-term care placement and over inability to care for the relative at home

- talk of role reversal or, more accurately, the filial crisis

- anger and resentment directed at the impaired relative

- embarrassment over the impaired relative's behavior

- concrete concerns about how to communicate with the demented person, about whether reality orientation works, and so forth

- painful losses as the impaired person declines and no longer recognizes family members.

Long-term care facilities are excellent settings for the formation of family support groups. A skilled group leader can assist families in working through this difficult time in the family life cycle and help families to establish realistic expectations of the impaired relative, of staff, and of themselves.

We offer monthly support groups. However, more intensive time-limited weekly groups that meet for 8 to 12 weeks are another option; the group can be designed to fit the needs of the families and facility involved.

Reference

Blenker, M. 1965. Social work and family relationships in later life with some thoughts on filial maturity. In *Social Structure and the Family: Generational Relations,* ed. by Shanas, Strieb, and Gorden. Englewood Cliffs, NJ: Prentice Hall.

Additional Reading

Aronson, M. D., and E. S. Yatzkan. 1984. Coping with Alzheimer's disease through support groups. *Aging* 347:3 -9.

Brody, E. M. 1972. Aging and family personality: A developmental view. Paper presented at the Conference on Loss, Death, Separation and the Family. Philadelphia: The Family Institute.

Carter, E., and M. McGoldrick. 1980. The Family Life Cycle: *A Framework for Family Therapy.* New York: Gardner Press.

Hausman, C. P. 1979. Short-term counseling groups for people with elderly parents. *Gerontologist* 19(1):102 - 107.

Maxey, L. B. 1981. Therapeutic interaction with families of the confused elderly. In *Confusion: Prevention and Care,* ed. by M. O. Wolanin and L. R. Fraelich-Phillips. St. Louis: C. V. Mosby Company.

McGoldrick, M., J. Pearce, and J. Giordano, eds. 1982. *Ethnicity and family therapy.* New York: Guilford Press.

Rhodes, S. M. 1977, May. A developmental approach to the life cycle of the family. *Social Casework:* 301 - 311.

Spark, G. M., and E. M. Brody. 1970. The aged are family members. *Family Process* 9(2):195 - 210.

Strow, C., and R. Mackreth. 1977. Family group meetings: strengthening a partnership. *Journal of Gerontological Nursing* 3(1):30 - 35.

Teusink, J. P., and S. Makler. Helping families cope with Alzheimer's disease. *Hospital and Community Psychiatry* 35(2):152 - 156.

Chapter 7

The Resource of Environmental Design

Passive and Active Design in Special Care Units*

Charles Silverman

For individuals undergoing the debilitating effects of dementia, the home environment—whether a personal home or a care facility—can become at once threatening and frustrating. Daily activities, once taken for granted, become insurmountably difficult; approaching the simplest of tasks causes such anxiety that the elderly eventually withdraw from all social intercourse.

One way to improve the impact of impairments due to Alzheimer's and related diseases is to provide an environment that is sensitive to the needs of both the resident and the staff.

Several key issues should be addressed:

- safety and security: the need to provide better observation and control of residents as they move about their unit

- orientation: the need to provide visual cues for the cognitively impaired

- emotional well-being: the need to reduce the anxiety of residents and provide social stimulation in their daily routines.

*While this chapter focuses on design considerations for special care units in long-term care facilities, families caring for Alzheimer's patients at home can adapt many of these features for home use.

Safety and Security

Staff needs are too often overlooked, especially in staff-intensive units for the care of impaired Alzheimer's patients. The setting has to provide a good working environment, but it also must remove physical constraints and improve observation and control. The goal is to achieve *passive design.*

Passive design provides a cost-effective, simple, common sense approach to relieving environmental problems without resorting to overly sophisticated equipment for monitoring activities.

- Consider the sightlines from a nursing station. Are they uninterrupted by walls or turns in corridors? Can staff observe the general activity as well as monitor exits?

- Consider the typical nursing station which is designed to above-waist height. Lowering the station to desk level allows better vision by staff, especially when sitting, and also improves resident and staff interaction.

- Consider how natural light enters an activity space or corridor. Sunlight, especially when low on the horizon, can backlight subjects so that it is difficult to distinguish persons or activities.

To promote these passive design goals, a facility can abandon the traditional skilled nursing unit layout with its double-loaded corridors for an open space concept (see Figure 1) that eliminates constraints imposed by corridors and corners.

This approach provides unlimited observation from the nursing station and optimizes utility of the corridor by incorporating it into an activity space. In addition, there is a potential for reducing the staff-to-patient ratio in a unit with a high staff intensity.

In skilled nursing facilities, smaller, more manageable special units, containing 25 to 30 beds, are recommended for the care of Alzheimer's patients.

The concept suggested in Figure 1 shows a 24-bed unit on either side of a nursing station. The design allows for segregation of patients

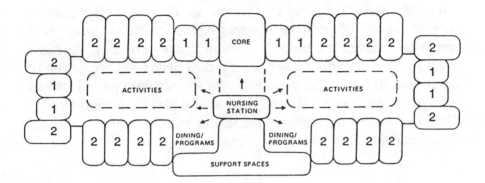

Figure 1. Open Space Concept

by behavior and function. The two 24-bed units, serviced by one central nursing station, offer obvious cost savings and staff efficiencies and yet provide direct service to each patient. The proposed scheme anticipates a staff-to-patient ratio of 1:4.8 during the day shift.

In an *active design* mode, electronic monitoring devices are employed. Closed circuit TV monitors make it possible to supervise corridors and spaces that are not readily observable. Potentials exist for providing residents with a greater degree of freedom of access. As an example, current technology has developed proximity detection devices that allow monitoring of individuals wearing ID cards that feature microcircuits imprinted with personalized codes. With the aid of a microcomputer, nurses determine and log the approximate location of each resident.

Orientation

Orientation is important to the cognitively impaired. Door numbers or directional signs, visual guideposts that we tend to take for granted, are of little use to such a patient. However, color coding of hallways and doors is useful to a confused patient trying to find his or her way. In Goldfine Pavilion at The Hebrew Home for the Aged at Riverdale, New York, patients' doors are decorated with graphic representations of personal mementos. An individual who loved music and played the piano in a more active period of life has a painting of keyboards on her door, a card player has a painting of cards, and so forth. These graphic symbols not only provide visual cues to orientation but also promote useful periods of reminiscing. Orientation is an important ingredient in reducing anxiety, thereby contributing to emotional well-being.

Emotional Well-Being

The home's environment should be nonagitative. Proper use of lighting, colors, and textures controls this problem. In institutional settings, too often fluorescent fixtures are used for their efficiency and low operating costs, but incandescent lighting has a more pleasing effect and is not as disturbing as fluorescence. Solid colors on walls and floors are less disturbing than stripes or complex patterns; a narrow-striped floor pattern, combined with fluorescent lighting can have a negative effect by creating the illusion of a tripping obstacle.

In the difficult area of providing daily activities, it is usually advisable to bring all patient activity programs directly to the care unit; this permits the resident to remain in a familiar environment and thereby lessens anxiety. A further benefit of on-site activities is that they provide more effective management and optimize staff use.

Program spaces can provide stimulation and reinforce patients' well-being. The space may be simply an observable multipurpose room with designated areas for a piano and other musical instruments and with adjacent space for dancing, or space can be designated as an indoor garden (with adjacent water supply) that can stimulate a productive avocation for residents. Developing a small zoo for keeping domesticated animals in a care unit has been suggested. Barring technical issues raised by health codes, this type of approach is well worth considering.

Designing a new special care unit may not be necessary. Adaptive reuse of existing facilities or units to meet the needs of Alzheimer's patients can be achieved with minimal cost. In a recent case study, The Hebrew Home for the Aged at Riverdale undertook the development of a special care unit (SCU) for the moderately to severely demented. The home neither built a new unit nor changed the basic floor plans, but creatively readapted the space to provide an environment that is protective, orienting, anxiety-reducing, and supportive of social activities. Changes included inexpensive orientation tools such as color coding doorways and corridors and affixing patient doors with representations of personal mementos.

For safety and security, the home added double-view mirrors to help staff better monitor the unit. The nurses' station was cut down to desk height level to promote better observation and provide ease of interaction between wheelchair-bound residents and staff. Programs were brought to the unit and used existing multipurpose space (dining area). The expense incurred to facilitate the unit was minimal but brought great improvements. Preliminary evaluation after four months indicated that patient anxiety levels had been reduced, the number of accidents had decreased, and there was a significant reduction in acting-out behavior by patients.

In the final analysis, the success of developing a well-designed special care unit relies on the philosophy and dedication of staff and their relationships to the patients. The environment simply provides a tool to help them more ably carry out their mission as caregivers.

Supportive Design For People With Memory Impairments

Lorraine G. Hiatt

Overview

There was a time when it seemed the only feature signifying an interest in design for people with mental impairments was a reality orientation board (Barns et al. 1973). The board lists facility name, date, and weather information. It was the unusually sensitive facility that took the concepts of reality therapy and integrated them with a more personal approach to memory development and design: personalized rooms, individualized door decorations or bedsides. Until recently, neither programs nor design have been clearly derived from research on mental impairment (Zeplin, Wolfe, and Kleinplatz 1981).

By the 1980s media attention (*Newsweek* 1984) and self-help groups such as the Alzheimer's Disease and Related Disorders Association (ADRDA) had given the sponsors of services for mentally impaired persons something they had never before had—consumer interest. As families read and became more involved in questions and interventions for mental impairment, they demanded more of long-term care institutional and day care providers. An educated public and the spirit of competition have fostered interest in environmental design. Environments communicate. At first, some sponsors look for environmental features to underscore their intent to serve mentally impaired persons. However, as one delves more deeply into the care of people with Alzheimer's type senile dementia or related diagnoses, it becomes increasingly clear that design is not an adjunct but at the heart of a full-service program.

Questions Illustrating the Interaction Between Program and Design

- Should we have a special unit?

  If so, who should be on it?

  If not, what are the alternatives?

- What group sizes are most appropriate?
- What should we do about wandering?
- What are the implications of grouping people of like abilities on a unit?
- What are the options for security at doors or elevators?
- How should color be used?
- What works best with orientation and way finding?
- What constitutes interior design for mentally impaired persons?
- Can environmental design help us with agitation?
- How can we incorporate environmental design in reminiscence groups?
- What aspects of environments are troubling?
- What about restraint use? Are there alternatives?

These questions are the basis for this chapter. Much of the information is directed toward those venturing into program development as well as design. The information can be applied either to existing facilities or new structures.

Sources of Information

This chapter is based on several sources of information: (1) current literature as cited; (2) personally conducted research including three studies of wandering behavior and one on program development and design for mentally impaired persons (Glassgote et al. 1977; Hiatt 1985; Snyder et al. 1978; Hiatt 1980c; Rosenfield 1978; Molberg 1977); (3) site visits to over 400 U.S. and Canadian long-term care institutions and day care centers; (4) experiences gained directing one of the pioneering programs serving mentally impaired persons at the Ebenezer Society in Minneapolis, Minnesota; (5) consultation to 40 groups on the development of programs and facilities for people with Alzheimer's type senile dementia or related diagnosis; and (6) participation in conferences on innovations in environmental design (Innovations 1986).

Step 1: Defining the Population in Functional Terms

Researchers have developed several functional definitions of dementia. These definitions are useful because they translate biochemical and physiological changes into the language of capabilities or impairments. Based on observation and on the literature, it may be helpful to translate the biomedical definitions into attributes:

- Attention span. Difficulties in focusing attention may be characteristic of early to late stages of the disease (Cohen and Wu 1980).

- Predictable behavior. Some individuals may exhibit unpredictable behavior or behavior uncharacteristic of their previous life styles (Morscheck 1984).

- Memory. One or more of the following aspects of memory may be reduced: memory for fact, for action, for social behavior and norms, or for emotion.

- Concepts of time. One or more of the following aspects of time perception may be confused: differentiation between day and night, awareness of actual or clock time, and ability to distinguish passing time (yesterday, today, tomorrow).

- Definition of self and identification of others.

- Physical skills including balance, swallowing, and control of body fluids.

- Concepts of space and location. Examples are: ability to identify present surroundings, follow directions, and formulate a mental map of a place.

Sometimes these notions are lumped together as *orientation;* however, that term seems unnecessarily broad (Hiatt 1985). This list may not be complete. The purpose of launching a design discussion with a functional profile of mental impairment is to provide a model that needs to be developed by each sponsor and updated with more specific information. Design should be based on knowledge of people and on a clear statement and schedule of the program or services to be offered. The description of people, sometimes called a functional profile, needs to clarify what individuals *can* as well as *cannot* do. This is the basis for planning a supportive environment.

A functional profile may contain data on older people that goes beyond the mental diagnosis and encompasses the whole person (Hiatt 1986a). Mobility, manual dexterity, sensitivity to odors, and responsiveness to touch are all useful descriptors. If most of the mentally impaired people who will use a program space have difficulty walking or use wheelchairs, we would want to design programs and facilities for their needs as well as for the needs of those who are ambulatory.

Step 2: Setting the Objectives

What can one expect from a well-designed environment? Environments and products or utensils may work together for the benefit of memory (Hiatt 1986b). Environments may:

- convey expectations and reinforce and elicit behavior
- improve attention span
- minimize agitation
- provide comfort and security
- prompt recollections or externalize memory
- cue behavior such as way finding
- reinforce concepts of time
- pique curiosity or stimulate alertness
- facilitate interpersonal relationships
- support emotional changes.

Mental impairment is probably not caused by environmental design. However, mental functioning may be facilitated by careful design planning. Some of the confused behavior exhibited by older people in the typical institutional environment may be magnified by inappropriately detailed physical and social environments. In a sense, environmental management may alleviate some excess disability (Brody et al. 1971) and allow the individual to function optimally within whatever residual capability he or she possesses.

A sponsor can address as many or as few of these objectives as imagination permits. As the following section will indicate, not all aspects of environmental design require financial investment.

Step 3: Identify the Attributes of Environments to be Addressed

At least four attributes of the environment need to be considered in planning supportive settings.

1. *The physical environment.* This refers to sights, sounds, textures, temperatures, air quality, space, and objects (Hiatt 1986b).

2. *The social environment.* Social environments encompass people: the number of individuals present, their roles and characteristics (mobility, alertness, activities, interactions, and positional relationships; i.e., near or far, standing or seated).

3. *The psychological environment.* Psychological environments are mental concepts of reality. Perceptions are influenced by vision, hearing, tactile sensitivity, speed of response, and the like (Fozard and Popkin 1979; Marsh 1980). Responses to the environment include perceptions (such as color), mental images (such as routes or relationships), and preferences (such as reactions to color or use of maps) (Moore and Golledge 1976).

4. *Norms and patterns.* Environments are also characterized by norms and patterns of use (Parr 1980). Some of the behavior problems attributed to older people may be rooted in long-practiced routines of caregivers. I visited one facility where wheelchairs were routinely issued to virtually everyone upon admission. Sometimes a single episode of wandering is dealt with by restraint forever thereafter (Burnside 1980). I have learned that innovation and change often involve rethinking such norms. A more encompassing example of the interaction between norms and environmental design for mentally impaired people is the notion that these people are too confused to know their surroundings. That concept may translate into policies that focus design on the most alert and provide the most institutional or sensory-deprived environments for cognitively impaired persons.

Dr. M. Powell Lawton was one of the first to question this chain of decisions. He asserts that the more impaired the individuals, the more significant the physical environment becomes to their level of competence (Lawton 1982; 1984).

By considering physical, social, and psychological attributes of environments, by reviewing norms, by taking stock of the local geography and culture, of the religious practices, size, and economic status of a home or day care program, it is possible to create a supportive environment in either new or vintage facilities.

Step 4: Match the Appropriate Population with Appropriate Design Focus

Experienced sponsors frequently think of mental impairment in terms of degree or stages (Mace and Rabins 1980). Some sponsors agonize over whether they should focus their programs on early, middle, or late stages of dementia (Innovations 1986). Design may offer a method of responding to a full continuum of capability and need.

Design and Early Stages

My colleagues and I have developed a set of instructional materials focused on early stages of sensory impairment and minor difficulties with memory. The package may be used in peer support groups or as self-help aids (Hiatt et al. 1982). The articles and discussion materials focus on methods of adapting environments or externalizing memory through props. Participants are urged to develop the social environment and each other's learning and response style. The material is based on the premise that if some older people could be freed from the anxiety surrounding memory impairment or could develop techniques for optimizing memory early in the aging process, such techniques might have value later on. Similar thinking is illustrated in the work of Zarit, Zarit, and Reever (1982); Zarit, Gallagher, and Kramer (1975) and of Perlmutter, Tenney, and Smith (1980), although those studies have not been as focused on the potential of the physical environment as a compensatory mechanism.

Design and Middle Stages

Most programs and special units appear to be focused on the middle stages of the disorder, characterized by more frequent impairments. The older people might have difficulty coping with life in an unsupervised environment or show sporadic problems in judgment. One controversy for some program sponsors has been whether middle stages are defined by loss of mobility. There has been a tendency to focus programs and special units on those who are ambulatory, relegating those in wheelchairs to a more traditional or even custodial care system. I am concerned that ambulation is an inappropriate differential diagnosis, especially when sedentary behavior may be induced by policy.

Design and Late Stages

Little has been published on appropriate models of care for people who are characterized by multiple mental and physical impairments and who may be unresponsive to group work. Based on my site visits and the lack of published information, it seems that the environments for these individuals have seldom been addressed. I would like to see greater attention paid to the lifespaces of severely impaired individuals: seating, beds, ceilings, clothing and footwear, lighting, odors, textures, and acoustics. The goal may be to contribute to the comfort of persons whose energy is too limited for other programs. Familiar surroundings may be superior to those filled exclusively with high tech, nontouch, unnameable machinery.

Continuity of care from initial to final stages of mental impairment has been lacking. Environmental design may prove a key to such continuity as certain features may offset the strangeness of technology or of unfamiliar caregivers.

Step 5: Tackle the Question of Special Units: Roles, Alternatives, and Implications

Increasingly, institutions and sponsors of day care are asking about the role of specially designated units. Some sponsors simply presume that separation and specialization are a prerequisite of service and design for mentally impaired persons.

Special units allow the organization to focus scarce resources on staff training, on a special group of people, and on an identifiable space. They give the service greater recognition value and with that may come prestige. In an existing facility, a special unit may be a way of saying "now we are doing something." A special unit may also allow a sponsor freedom to improvise and to deviate from traditional methods of service delivery, offering more meals or nighttime programs, for example.

The question of whether there is value in isolating mentally impaired persons from their peers has not been well researched and continues to be controversial. Most sponsors presume that separation benefits the alert and adept, although there have been at least two studies that suggest that some alert people thrive on comingling

(Salsbury and Goehner 1983; Hiatt 1984). Special units need not mean that all people are of one level of mental functioning nor that all groups or socializing occurs with people of the same degree of alertness.

The question of grouping might better be based upon sleep cycles, sensitivity to verbalization, activity patterns, personalities, programs, or staffing. Ideally, families might become more adept at selecting from a variety of social and physical contexts those most in keeping with the behavioral needs of the older person.

Caution—separating by ability does not constitute a program! The fact that a unit is provided for people of similar diagnoses, even if a few extra hours of traditional nursing assistance are added, does not necessarily mean that special services are also provided. I have toured special units where motion is controlled (through the use of geriatric wheelchairs and restraints) and where boredom is rampant; fragmented behavior is tolerated, and normal stimuli and institutional activities are limited.

What are some of the considerations that have led sponsors to phase out or adopt alternatives to special units? Some facilities are too small or do not lend themselves architecturally to specialization. Some day care programs are too small, or the families that utilize them cannot agree on one time period for a particular kindred group. Special units presume that someone is skilled at identifying people who have Alzheimer's disease. As of this writing, viable diagnoses are still deductions based upon ruling out other factors (see Chapter Three; Jarvik 1980). Policies and norms regarding special units may presume that people do not change; they do. Special units may isolate staff on that unit from their peers and require special measures to overcome the feeling of extra burden that may result. Special units may become unduly enclosed and confining to either residents or staff. Many of these issues may be resolved with adequate advance planning or continuous and sensitive management.

There are alternatives to separate units. The Masonic Home of Wallingford, Connecticut, and Villa Maria Nursing Home, Fargo, North Dakota, have developed in-house day care programs. People from different parts of the building come together for special services catering to their needs and strengths. Design resources are focused on one room serving some people for an hour and others for longer stretches. An off-unit program was developed in conjunction with a special unit by Sawyer and Mendlovitz (1982; 1984).

For some sponsors, separate units are a phase in development. The sponsor begins to ask, "What am I doing on this unit that does not apply to the full population?" With nursing home clientele becoming increasingly frail and the public developing a concern over the inadequacies of custodial care, what is special about separate units may be that some energy is being focused on a population formerly omitted from socialization and intervention. The foregoing suggests that we be cautious in naming a unit. "Special unit" should not come to mean that older people (or staff) outside its parameters are somehow less than special. Perhaps terms such as "kindred" unit, "AllsHome" ("Alzhome"), or "The Elizabeth Seton Center" are all more apropos.

Step 6: Develop a Personal Design Agenda

Good design transcends the decision to create separate units or programs. Most of these considerations have applicability in institutions and day care settings; some also apply to people in households. A list such as this may be used as a guide; sponsors may adapt the concepts or create their own examples.

- Alleviate problem stimuli.

    Example: Minimize noxious background noise, glare, shadow, and dimness.

    Reason: Such stimuli dissipate attention.

- Expand the potential of the sensory environment.

    Example: Increase lighting on tasks that require concentration: eating, dressing, and transactions.

Reason: By meeting basic functional needs for more lighting, it is possible to focus attention.

- Minimize sensory overload (Lawton 1982).

    Example: Multiple competing stimuli are those that demand attention but cannot be simultaneously heeded: sounds from two or more sources, music during conversation, pedestrian traffic during group meetings.

    Reason: When sensory input competes for attention, it may overload the system and fragment behavior or frustrate the individual attempting to respond.

- Stimulate the sense of touch and the need to clutch (Hiatt 1980c).

    Example: Develop human contact as culturally appropriate through back rubs, foot massage, hand lotion, scalp massage, and the like. Consider children and pets as tactile resources. Provide touchable objects within reach: finger foods, clothing, footwear, and bath aids. Texturally engaging activities include bathing, cooking, baking, gardening, or manipulating heated soil.

    Reason: Humans appear to have a basic need for tactile stimulation that is sustained despite cognitive impairments. Tactile stimulation may also minimize agitation, provide comfort, and reduce excessive verbalization (calling out).

Note: Textural stimulation may also be beneficial for bedridden mentally impaired persons.

- Provide environmental features supportive of emotional outbursts.

  Example: What can be tugged, dug, torn, socked, smashed, stuck underfoot, thwarted, or squeezed? An outside area for digging (rather than gardening), pillows that need fluffing, a punching bag or squirt gun may each have some proponents. Ask family about former methods of sloughing off anger and consider how these may be safely transferred to the health care environment.

  Reason: Demented individuals need acceptable means of venting anger. Some may find nonverbal methods more satisfying and workable than verbalization.

- Create programs and environments, and select furnishings that engage people in exercise.

  Example: Provide access to fresh air and walks, and install furniture that bounces, rocks, or swivels safely.

  Reason: Exercise is important to overall physical functioning and also may prove beneficial to mental responses and emotional well-being (Posner et al. 1986). Exercise may also stave off some of the agitation associated with wandering (Hiatt 1985).

- Develop a specific program for orientation to place that can enable users to build up way-finding skills (Hiatt 1980a).

Example: Actual experience—seeing the building from the outside, approaching from many angles—can be helpful in spatial orientation (Weisman 1986). Name rooms and halls with familiar terms. Link names with landmarks or geography rather than obscuring them in the jargon of health care. Use the names in conversation, written materials, and signs. Couple meaningful objects with significant places. Real objects may be more helpful than abstract graphics or symbols. These landmarks need to be detectable from a distance. Name plates may be useful as verification when one is in front of a doorway. Volunteers or staff in an institution may be the best, most believable sources of information.

Reason: Landmarks and practice may facilitate way finding and comfort those who are concerned about being lost or who are proud of their independence. Research on spatial orientation suggests that some people have never had good directional sense (Blasch and Hiatt 1983). Way finding refers to the ability to get to a predetermined destination using a planned and efficient method. Places are more difficult to image or locate when they have unclear names or when names are not coordinated with signs.

- To minimize problem rummaging, camouflage features that should not attract the attention of the curious.

  Example: This may involve use of nondistinguishable colors and hidden doors or latches. Camouflaging is not likely to be distracting if there are at the same time appropriate, interesting places for an individual to satisfy the needs of rummaging and exploration (Hiatt 1981). Caution: exit doors should not be so well disguised that fire or life safety measures are compromised. Individuals may need to feel that they can get out and are not incarcerated.

Reason: Out of sight, out of mind.

- Create a range of social contexts or settings.

    Example: The environment as a whole might consist of private spaces, spaces for dyads or intimacy, spaces for family-sized groups, for classroom-sized groups, and for full assembly (DeLong 1970; Snyder 1978; Hiatt 1983; Pastalan 1986).

    Reason: Each individual typically needs some "time out" and some time in the company of others. Individuals and caregivers can often benefit from 15 to 45 minutes off the unit or away from a fragmented social situation.

- Carefully consider the group size in which the individual functions best.

    Example: Develop ways of working with small groups, perhaps six to eight rather than 25 to 40 persons. This can be especially useful in reminiscence groups and in dining, where the distractions of many other individuals may interrupt dining or self-feeding. Families may also be guided during visits to respond to appropriate group considerations.

Reason: Crowding or density may be problematic for some impaired older people. Too many people, especially too many similarly impaired people, may contribute to heightened confusion for all.

- Use objects and possessions to cue and evoke behavior.

Example: Personal objects from familiar possessions to sounds, smells, and images may stimulate memory and encourage thinking. Use objects and decorative features to extend the value of color in evoking responses and creating a mood (Hiatt 1980b).

Note: The environment needs to afford a safe place to hang, display, or keep the objects. High shelves, tackable walls, or glass cases are all possible locations for keeping items available yet safe. Encourage areas where exhibits of objects may be presented and may change regularly—unlike landmarks, which should be stable and predictable.

- Select objects that have familiar intuitive operation wherever possible.

Example: Eating utensils of familiar weight such as ceramic cups and metal forks may be easier to clutch than styrofoam and plastic. For particularly demanding activities of daily living, consider the use of tools with familiar ways of operating. Dial clocks and phones may work better for some than do digital ones; toilets with a conventionally placed handle are more likely to be flushed. Pull cords may be easier to use than push button call systems.

Reason: Certain operations may have become nearly mindless; the person may not be able to verbalize steps, but may recall how to manage familiar and repeated operations. Telephones, steering wheels, and even a stick shift may all be somewhat familiar to some older people whereas keypads, single control faucets, and digital radios may require not only learning new ways but also unlearning long-held notions.

Note: There is a role for specially designed objects, such as those that make eating easier for one with palsy or impaired grip, but search for implements that do not challenge long-held process memories and that look relatively familiar.

- Develop the potential for rooms, outdoor places, or attributes of the environment that can help people shift moods or lift spirits, using environmental change to provide a spiritual vacation.

Example: Vary room decor, smell, and lighting from one space to another. In institutions, some of the spaces that can be developed for these purposes are bedrooms (for solitude), parlors and living rooms (for action and socialization); hallways (for exercise and perhaps manual exploration of a tactile museum or memory lane); courtyards and secure but unusually shaped outdoor areas (for meandering and visiting); and bathing rooms (that can be far less institutional and more relaxing through the use of familiar objects, textural variety, color accents, and vestibular stimulation) (Snyder 1978; Hiatt 1980b, 1983).

Reason: People of many ages use a change of surroundings to stimulate fresh thinking. The environment may reach a person who does not respond
to group work or to other direct communications.

- Take advantage of natural inclinations and remembered response.

Example: Many confused persons respond to odors: yeast
breads, cocoa, familiar spices, popcorn, and so
on. Often odors are masked by body processes,
by smelly pharmaceuticals, and by housekeeping supplies that are thought to clean better the
stronger they smell.

Reason: It may be useful to the person's overall self-
concept and comfort level as well as to the
reactions of caregivers to identify and satisfy
residual memory or responses.

- Reinforce a positive self-image.

Example: Photographs and sounds may be useful in put-
ting people back in touch with themselves.
Illustrations on beauty shop walls that show a
range of beautiful older women (including
residents), hair decorations, or grooming de-
canters may all contribute to a sense of beauty.
Other reinforcements to positive self-images
include use of artwork or visuals combined
with music, sounds and textures or scenarios of
intergenerational life, humor, powerful emotions, cultural attachments (patriotism, faith,
healing, liturgy), and local pride. Such props
may also be the focus of group work or
informal memory development.

Reason: Orientation to self may be one of the functional losses associated with severe mental impairment. In early stages of memory loss, some self-confidence may be lost as well, contributing to depressive states. In the latter stages, a positive self-image may be as helpful to reinforce the efforts of caregivers as it is to the overall well-being of the individual.

Note: The environment needs to emphasize these items. Select colors or background materials that draw attention to the significance of personal possessions and people. Some wall coverings are so vivid that they dwarf the significance of either people or their possessions. Be cautious with the placement of mirrors. Mirrors should be in grooming areas or above mantels and in general should not be used as wall decor where they may be mistaken for windows or otherwise be disorienting.

Step 7: Rethink the Approach to Wandering

There are probably different types of wandering (Hiatt 1985), each of which warrants a different form of intervention. In a study of 170 institutions randomly selected from eight states across the United States, I learned that most institutional caregivers may anticipate wandering and then attempt to develop a single set of solutions to work throughout an institution or day care center. The irony is that most directors of nursing indicated that they are implementing interventions which, in their judgment, do not work well. In case study work, it appears that exercise, provision of energy outlets, and enriched activity may assist many wanderers. For others, the motion is itself therapeutic and warrants finding appropriate places where people may exercise.

Some facilities, such as the Motion Picture and Television Studio Retirement Center in Woodland Hills, California, have set up wandering gardens to create unusually configured environments for those who enjoy motion. We need to develop these types of gardens indoors. Others have developed runaway drills, provided practice sessions, offered opportunities for wanderers to tag along, and increased the availability of orienting landmarks to help wanderers who are also disoriented.

Step 8: Review the Approach to Controls and Restraints

Recent research in nursing has suggested that we rethink the issue of restraint use for older people (Nordstrom et al. 1983). A growing body of research suggests that motion is important to behavior (Posner et al. 1986). Nordstrom and others suggest that if a patient is restrained because he or she wanders, the person "may be in less danger if allowed to wander than if restrained . . ." and that even if the person is restrained to prevent falls, "it would be wiser to risk the fall than to restrain without observation" (1983: 136). Another nursing study indicated that caregivers often restrain out of habit and may not know why restraints were first ordered for long-stay patients (Robb et al. 1985). In my own research on wandering, 82 percent of the institutions used body holders or geriatric wheelchairs, with 45 percent of respondents using both geriatric wheelchairs and restraints for wanderers, 19 percent using body holders only, and 18 percent using geriatric wheelchairs only (Hiatt 1985: 184).

How might a caregiver reduce restraint use? The process may take several months or even more than a year. Try to use some of these methods that have been employed in facilities with which I have worked.

- Review when restraints are used, on whom, and why.

- Develop a plan and policy of risk reduction so that nursing assistants do not bear full responsibility for decisions. Engage families in discussions and consider methods of involving them in searches for alternatives (Snyder et al. 1978; Hiatt 1985).

- Minimize environmental hazards related to falling: poor lighting, poorly selected chairs, obstacles in the environment, and the like.

- Make sure there are study chairs and platform rockers available and consider the use of conventional wheelchairs with and without tray tables. Chairs should be measured to fit the individual. Feet should be supported, and the individual should be free to move about in the chair.

- Implement effective bowel and bladder training programs (need for a bathroom may be a factor in attempts to fight restraints or bedrails).

- Reevaluate medications and consider their role in risks of falls.

- Develop body strength through an appropriate, medically indicated program of exercise including chair exercises.

- Secure the range of risky boundaries, perhaps through telemetric technologies such as selective security systems.

- Analyze management reasons for, and patterns of staffing that are associated with higher utilization of restraint use; develop better methods of coping with these difficulties.

- If restraints are to be reduced, start slowly and work with people in whom staff and families have confidence.

Restraint reduction may not work for everyone, though there have been institutions that have less than 1 percent of a skilled care population utilizing restraints. The institution that trades physical restraints for pharmacological ones probably has not improved the situation.

Final Thoughts

Design cannot precede program. Whether a sponsor is involved with new construction or with an existing facility, the best design is one that fits the functional definition of the population and is responsive to the services and local geography. I doubt there will ever be one perfect design or model unit. We need many models: programs for small retirement centers, for large, specialized units, and for integrated ones. We need service and design combinations that will work in acute care as well as in residential settings.

No one single decor or prototype of furnishings can satisfy all impaired older people. Though we may start with a common methodology or some agreement regarding the potential of environmental design, the look can be as distinctive as one likes. As corporations become increasingly involved in long-term care, I do become a bit concerned that we will attempt to legislate one model concept.

My travels have taught me that there are many good and right ways of designing for mentally impaired persons. The wrong approach is to dress up the unit without meeting the individuals' underlying needs and potential. Care of people with Alzheimer's disease or related diagnoses is a key factor in the transition from custodialism or high quality, but passive, care to more meaningful intervention for all recipients of long-term care.

References

Barns, E. K., A. Sack, and H. Shore. 1973. Guidelines to treatment approaches. *Gerontologist* 11(4):513 - 537.

Blasch, B., and L. G. Hiatt. 1983. *Orientation and way finding*. Technical paper. Washington, DC: Architectural and Transportation Barriers Compliance Board.

Brody, E. M. et al. 1971. Excess disability of mentally impaired aged. Impact of individualized treatment. *Gerontologist* 11(2):124 - 132.

Burnside, I. 1980. *Psychosocial Nursing Care of the Aged.* 2d ed. New York: McGraw Hill: 298 - 309.

Cohen, D., and S. Wu. 1980. Language cognition during aging. In C. Eisdorfer, ed. *Annual Review of Gerontology and Geriatrics.* New York: Springer: 71 - 96.

DeLong, A. J. 1970. The micro-spatial behavior of the older person: Some implications of planning the social and spatial environment. In L. A. Pastalan and D. H. Carson, eds., *Spatial Behavior of Older People.* Ann Arbor: University of Michigan: 25 - 39.

Fozard, J. L., and S. J. Popkin. 1979. Optimizing adult development: Ends and means of an applied psychology of aging. *American Psychologist* 33:975 - 989.

Glassgote, E., J. E. Gudeman, and D. Miles. 1977. *Creative Mental Health Services for the Elderly.* Washington, DC: Joint Information Services of the American Psychiatric Association.

Hiatt, L. G. 1981. Color and care: The selection and use of colors in environments for older people. *Nursing Homes* 30 (3):18 - 22.

_____. 1980a. Disorientation is more than a state of mind. *Nursing Homes* 29(4):30 - 36.

_____. 1983. Effective design for informal conversation. *American Health Care Association Journal* 9(2):43 - 46.

_____. 1986a. Environmental design and mentally impaired older people. In H. Altman, ed., *Alzheimer's Disease: Problems, Prospects and Perspectives.* New York: Plenum, in press.

_____. 1986b. The environment's role in the total well-being of the older person. In *Well-Being and the Elderly: An Holistic View,* ed. by G. G. Magan and E. L. Haught. Washington, DC: American Association of Homes for the Aging: 23 - 38.

_____. 1980b. The happy wanderer. *Nursing Homes* 29(2):27 - 31.

_____. 1980c. Touchy about touching. *Nursing Homes* 29(6):42 - 46.

_____. 1984. Understanding the physical environment. *Pride Institute Journal of Long-Term Health Care* 4(2): 12- 22.

_____. 1985. Wandering behavior of older people. Doctoral dissertation, Graduate Center, City University of New York. *1985 Dissertation Abstracts International* 46. University Microfilms No. 86-01:653.

Hiatt, L. G. et al. 1982. *What are friends for? Self-help groups for older persons with sensory loss.* New York: American Foundation for the Blind.

Innovations in care of the memory impaired elderly. June 11 - 23, 1986. A national conference sponsored by the New York State Department of Health. New York: Proceedings forthcoming.

Jarvik, L. 1980. Diagnosis of dementia in the elderly: A 1980 perspective. In *Annual Review of Gerontology and Geriatrics* 1, ed. by C. Eisdorfer: 180 - 203.

Lawton, M. P. 1982. Competence, environmental press and the adaptation of older people. In *Aging and the Environment*, ed. by M. P. Lawton, P. Windley, and T. Byerts. New York: Springer: 35 - 59.

_____. 1984. An introduction and overview to environment. Pride Institute Journal of Long-Term Health Care 4:1 - 11.

Mace, N., and P. Rabins. 1980. *The 36-hour day.* Baltimore: Johns Hopkins University.

Marsh, G. R. 1980. Perceptual changes with age. In *Handbook of Geriatric Psychiatry,* ed. by E. W. Busse and D. G. Blazer. New York: Van Nostrand: 147 - 168.

Molberg, A. L. 1977, December. Catching-up. *Mental Health*: 11 - 13.

Moore, G. T., and R. G. Golledge, eds. 1976. Environmental knowing: Concepts and theories. In *Environmental Knowing*. Stroudsburg, PA: Dowden, Hutchinson & Ross: 3 - 26.

Morscheck, P. 1984. Introduction: An overview of Alzheimer's disease and long term care. *Pride Institute Journal of Long-Term Health Care* 3(4):4 - 10.

Nordstrom, M., D. L. Smith, and D. Meilicke. 1983. Monitoring elderly patients in restraints: Nursing practice, staffing and policy implications. *Proceedings of the First National Conference on Gerontological Nursing*. Victoria, B.C.: University of Victoria Extension Conference Office: 131 - 136.

Parr, J. 1980. The interaction of persons and living environments. In *Aging in the 1980s,* ed. by L. Poon. Washington, DC: American Psychological Association: 393 - 406.

Pastalan, L. 1986. Six principles for a caring environment. *Provider* 12 (4):4 - 5.

Perlmutter, L. C., Y. Tenney, and P. Smith. 1980. *The evaluation and remediation of memory problems in the aged.* Boston: Veterans Administration Outpatient Memory and Learning Clinic.

Posner, J. D., et al. 1986. Exercise in the elderly. *American Journal of Cardiology* 57 (5):52c - 58c.

Robb, S. S. et al. 1985. *Restraint usage in long-term care.* Pittsburgh: VA Medical Center Research Committee Report.

Rosenfield, A. 1978. *New views on older lives.* Rockville, MD: National Institute of Mental Health.

Salsbury, S., and E. Goehner. 1983. Separation of the confused or integration with the lucid. *Geriatric Nursing* 4:231 - 233.

Sawyer, J., and A. Mendlovitz. 1984. Alzheimer's program progress report. San Antonio, TX: Paper presented at the 1984 Annual Meeting, American Association of Homes for the Aging.

_____. 1982, November. A management program for ambulatory institutionalized patients with Alzheimer's disease and related disorders. Boston: Paper presented at the annual meeting of the Gerontological Society.

Snyder, L. H. 1978. Environmental changes for socialization. *Journal of Nursing Administration* 8(1):44 - 50.

Snyder, L. H., et al. 1978. Wandering. *Gerontologist* 18, (3): 491 - 495.

Weisman, J. 1986. Way-finding and architectural legibility: Design considerations in housing environments. In *Housing for the Elderly: Satisfaction and Preferences,* ed. by V. Regnier and J. Pynoos. New York: Elsevier.

Zarit, S. H., D. Gallagher, and N. Kramer. 1975. Memory training in community aged: Effects on depression, memory complaint, and memory performance. *Educational Gerontology* 30:67 - 73.

Zarit, S. H., J. Zarit, and K. Reever. 1982. Memory training for severe memory loss: Effects on senile dementia patients and their families. *Gerontologist* 22(4):373 - 377.

Zeplin, H., C. S. Wolfe, and F. Kleinplatz. 1981. Reality orientation. *Journal of Gerontology* 31(1):70 - 77.

Additional Reading

Alzheimer's disease. 1981. A mini-conference report of the White House Conference on Aging. Washington, DC: U.S. Government Printing Office.

Grossman et al. 1985. The milieu standard for care of dementia in a nursing home. *Journal of Gerontological Social Work in Alzheimer's Disease*: Winter, 73 - 89.

Hiatt, L. G. 1982a. Grouping elders of different abilities. In *Congregate Housing for Older People: Preferences and Satisfactions,* ed. by R. D. Chellis and J. F. Seagle. Lexington, MA: Lexington/DC Heath.

Lindsley, O. 1964. Geriatric behavioral prosthetics. In *New Thoughts on Old Age,* ed. by R. Kastenbaum. New York: Springer: 41 - 60.

Mace, N. 1984. Report of a survey of day care centers. *Pride Institute Journal of Long-Term Health Care* 3(4):38 - 43.

Snyder, L. H. 1975. Living environments, geriatric wheelchairs, and older persons' rehabilitation. *Journal of Gerontological Nursing* 1(5):17 - 20.

Chapter 8

Care in the Community

Adult Day Care Within the Long-term Care Facility

Joan Scharf

As nursing homes expand into community-based services, adult day care is one of the services most frequently considered. Can a nursing home derive real benefits from including an adult day care program in its facility? How difficult is the task of developing such a service?

Four benefits that Menorah Park Center for the Aging in Beachwood, Ohio, has realized include positive public relations, preparation for nursing home placement, support to those on the waiting list, and a resource for the nursing home.

Positive Public Relations

Day care's foremost goal is to help families avoid unnecessary or premature placement by providing respite and support to caregivers and by helping to maintain the impaired person in the community at his or her maximum level of functioning. A recently completed evaluation of Menorah Park's Adult Day Care Program revealed that 60 percent of the caregivers felt day care had helped them avoid placement. As one caregiver stated, "This program saved my life. I am not ready to give my Mom up, and this program lifted a rock from my heart."

165

Fifty percent of the caregivers felt their family's overall functioning had been maintained, and an additional 40 percent felt their family member had actually improved. Only 10 percent felt there had been a decline. Participants' responses revealed an even greater perception of improved overall functioning. Two-thirds of the participants felt they had improved, one-third felt they had maintained their current functioning, and none felt there had been a decline. These statistics are nothing short of miraculous considering the reality of decline that staff anticipates and sees cognitively and physically, both in the Alzheimer's population and in those physically disabled with stroke, multiple sclerosis, and Parkinson's disease. Day center programs are succeeding in maintaining or improving these participants' social and emotional well-being which in turn contributes to an overall sense of improved functioning.

Preparation for Placement in the Nursing Home

The day center serves as a transitional experience. Typically, it provides a group program with congregate meals and some shared activity with residents in a nursing home setting. Participation in the day care center creates a positive identification with the long-term care facility. In our evaluation questionnaires, 50 percent of caregivers felt that day care participation had made it easier for them to consider or act upon the need to place their family member.

Support for Waiting List

If your nursing home is fortunate enough (or unfortunate enough, as the case may be) to have a waiting list, the day center can provide support to both caregiver and participant during the interim period. As placement approaches, the professional day care staff can provide counseling support to both family and participant. Often, involving the peer group of participants in support can be a critical factor in easing a person's acceptance of placement.

Facility Resource

The day center can serve as a resource for the long-term care facility. The day center can experiment with new approaches and programming. Typically, adult day care uses a psychosocial model with health care components. It can provide a model for the nursing units. Day care staff can serve as consultants; the program can serve as a training site for nursing unit staff. Moreover, leading a small group in the day center can provide nursing home staff with both stimulus and relief, for the day care center usually includes a higher functioning population than does the nursing home.

An important advantage of housing the adult day center within the long-term care facility is the potential savings in cost per person made possible by in-kind contributions of maintenance, housekeeping, bookkeeping staff, and administration.

What are some of the practical aspects of developing an adult day care center?

- The day center must be a self-contained unit so that participants do not infringe on the rights of the nursing home population.

- The day center must have its own entrance, eating, lounging, and activity space, bathrooms, pantry, and a small rest area.

- It must have its own staff.

- Transportation must be available.

For specific suggestions and requirements, refer to "Standards for Adult Day Care," published by the National Institute of Adult Day Care of the National Council on Aging.

Critical to developing an adult day care center is defining the reciprocal roles and responsibilities of the nursing home administration and department heads vis-a-vis the day care staff. Ideally, the executive director of the long-term care facility schedules individual meetings of the day care director with each department head in order to develop an operational understanding between the two departments. The understandings become written policy, reviewed and modified as necessary. Operational understandings should be developed with the medical director and with the nursing, activity, social and rehabilitation services, housekeeping, maintenance, dietary, and bookkeeping departments.

Once the proper groundwork is laid, a marketing program can help adult day care reach the community-based population. This population is in great need of services to help avoid or postpone premature nursing home placements. Who can provide this service better than the long-term care facility skilled in working with the impaired elderly population?

Adult Day Care for the Dementia Patient

Gloria Levine

Rationale

In 1982, the staff of the Menorah Park Adult Day Care Program began to see an increase in the number of persons concerned about family members with dementia who were participating in the day care program. The management of the dementia clients was a problem. The staff decided to initiate a small demonstration program for a group diagnosed as having Alzheimer's disease or a related disorder. They were ambulatory, could follow one- and two-step directions, and had moderate to severe language disturbances. Staff made use of activities such as art, dance, music, reading, cognitive stimulation, and group therapy; they also provided individual and family counseling.

The special programming improved patient management. It was concluded that with a separate self-contained unit, more staff, and more activities, a new specialized program for persons with dementia could be developed that could help maintain the family structure, delay institutionalization, and provide respite for the family. We submitted a proposal to the Cleveland Foundation and were awarded a three-year grant for a demonstration program. The Memory Impaired Day Care Program for Adults opened at Menorah Park in August 1983.

Goals

The goals of the program are to:

- maintain the mental and physical functioning of the patient
- encourage socialization and appropriate behavior
- enhance self-esteem

- provide respite for the caregiver
- provide support to patients and families to help them adapt to the patient's decline.

Intake

We require interviews with the potential patient and the patient's primary caregiver prior to admission to the program. The interviews are done separately by the program director, who is a registered nurse with a B.S. in nursing. A separate interview gives the caregiver freedom to express his or her feelings and concerns. Counseling often begins in the initial interview because of the caregiver's tremendous need to be listened to and to receive information and guidance.

In the patient's interview, the program director assesses mental and physical functioning, develops a trusting working relationship, and seeks information about the patient's feelings about life and about the memory problem. The director undertakes a careful evaluation to determine the extent and nature of intellectual decline. Acceptance into the program is based upon the individual's remaining skills and whether they are sufficient to allow successful participation in the program. The skills considered are:

- communication: degree of language disturbance. The patient must be able to communicate needs and to respond at least nonverbally.
- ability to follow one- or two-step directions.
- appropriate behavior: behavior must not be harmful to self or others or disruptive to group activity.
- appropriate language: frequent use of foul language is not acceptable.
- independent ambulation.
- continence of bowel.

Following completion of the evaluation, the director discusses a treatment plan with the caregiver and with the patient if appropriate. A medical information form is sent to the patient's private physician.

Program

In a day care center for people with cognitive and memory problems, it is important to keep the patient's days of attendance consistent and to provide a secure environment with a constant staff. Routine helps reduce anxiety in these patients.

A typical day begins at 9:30 a.m. with coffee and social conversation. At 10:15, the morning schedule begins with orientation and cognitive and memory stimulation (reminiscence, current events), followed by an activity such as music, movement or exercise, arts and crafts, and watching the noon news on television. There is a 45-minute lunch and relaxation period.

The afternoon schedule varies but always includes three of the following activities: art, dance, music, cognitive and physical games, walk, discussion, and special programs offered by the Menorah Park Activity Department. This population can handle selected large group events because the program staff always accompanies them. Wrap-up at 2:45 p.m. is a review of the day's activities and events.

Primary activities in which all patients take part are cognitive and memory stimulation and reminiscence, physical activity, and social interaction. Cognitive and memory stimulation and reminiscence are accomplished by the daily use of orientation. A blackboard carries information about the day's schedule, the patients, and staff. A large clock and calendar relate the time and date and a tagboard wall gives information and pictures. Staff frequently remind patients about the date, time, and names of staff and other patients. Reminiscence is stimulated by means of the creative arts therapies: art, music, dance, and pet therapy. Participation in number and word games, cooking, and horticulture allows patients not only to practice sequencing and object identification but also to be motivated to use past skills and activities.

All group members are encouraged to participate in a 30-minute physical activity period daily.

Staff reinforce appropriate social behavior throughout the day's activities. Appropriate communication and conversation are encouraged throughout the day, appropriate table manners are encouraged at lunch and snack times. Carefully selected, goal-oriented field trips have helped the group in the areas of reminiscence, cognitive and memory stimulation, and socialization.

The goal of the program is to meet the patient's human needs, build and maintain self-esteem, and provide meaningful activity, social interaction, and private space. Staff encourage patients to participate at their optimal levels, and staff acknowledge the individual accomplishments of the patients. Independence and peer help are also encouraged. Flexibility is incorporated into the programming to offer patients some control over their lives.

Staff

The Memory Impaired Adult Day Care Program includes the following full-time staff: the director, who has a bachelor's degree in nursing, two health assistants, and a part-time activity specialist. Assistants must be stable, mature, flexible, and able to relate to and care for others. The staff-to-patient ratio is approximately one to three. Volunteers help with activities such as art, music, exercise, and physical games.

Patient Grouping

Homogeneous grouping is a *must* to maintain a calm, therapeutic environment. Patients assessed with moderate dementia become very anxious and stressed when mixed with others who are more cognitively impaired. They feel threatened, express fear ("Is this going to happen to me?"), and withdraw from activity participation. Understandably, they become very upset with the inappropriate behavior of those more impaired. If seated by more impaired persons, they will actually get up and move. All of these feelings and reactive behaviors are very disruptive to programming.

Conversely, patients assessed as having severe dementia become very anxious and stressed when mixed with people more capable in cognitive function. The pressures of preserving their dignity, trying to perform tasks they can no longer perform, and participating in appropriate social interactions are so great that their anxiety escalates to heights that produce agitation and highly inappropriate behavior.

Severe language disturbance is equally difficult for both groups to cope with and accept. Visual and hearing impairments also affect how a person functions in a group; patients with a hearing impairment, for example, may not hear directions or may think people are talking to them and answer for others. Patients with visual impairments can have hallucinations because objects seem distorted; they receive benefit from visual cues in the environment.

Family's Support

In addition to providing a day care program for patients, we provide family members with knowledge, support, and techniques for coping with the stresses resulting from the patient's illness.

One vehicle for working with family members is the monthly caregivers' support group meeting. Co-led by the day care center director who has a master's degree in social work and the program director who has a nursing degree, it provides a forum for solving problems, sharing management techniques, identifying and dealing with feelings, and educating and informing. Formal and informal counseling with individual caregivers provides opportunities to work on management problems, family problems related to the stress of coping with the patient's decline, and future care planning.

Individual therapy with patients has been attempted; however, it only helps for the moment. There is very little, if any, carryover after the session. In only one instance has family therapy including both the caregiver and the patient provided the opportunity for problem management, discussion, and the sharing of feelings and emotions.

Evaluation

In an effort to determine the effect of our program on the natural course of the disease, we evaluate patients at regular intervals. By utilizing the Haycox Dementia Behavior Scale, we can measure functioning in the areas of language, social interaction, attention awareness, spatial orientation, motor coordination, bowel and bladder, eating and nutrition, and dressing and grooming. Numerical scores are plotted and changes in behavior and intellect are graphically visible. We ask families to respond to a program evaluation questionnaire after the patient has been in the program for three months.

Day care will not halt or change the progressive decline in the patient with dementia; it can, however, assist patients and families to cope with the decline. It can provide respite and help keep a family together. For many, day care can be a positive community-based alternative to premature nursing home placement.

Chapter 9

Conclusion

Jacob Reingold

In this concluding chapter, I want to return to Marion Roach's eloquent and poignant introduction.

Marion Roach's mother lives in the home of which I am executive vice president, and I am, of course, touched by the kindness of Marion's words. But there are many other nursing homes where men and women like Mrs. Roach are being well cared for, and there are thousands of children like Marion and her sister who are grateful for this care.

Rather, the point is in the last sentence of Marion's introduction: "My hope is that everyone with Alzheimer's can be enabled to have that kind of care, that quality of care." We now must turn to the realization of Marion's hope, for it was this hope that impelled Stephen L. Schwartz, president of The Brookdale Foundation, to underwrite the publication of this volume. The book represents also the hopes and intentions of the American Association of Homes for the Aging and the distinguished authors who contributed chapters to it. Now the questions we have to answer have to do with the future: how can we ensure that all of the Mrs. Roaches of our nation will receive the quality of care that they need and to which they are entitled? And how can we make certain that the families of Alzheimer's patients receive the help they need in facing one of the

175

cruelest fates that blights the lives of so many loving and responsible spouses and children?

We must begin with the painful recognition that although we hope that Burton Reifler's prediction "... that within the next decade we will see greatly improved treatment of Alzheimer's disease ..." will prove to be the case, research findings are not likely to be of more than marginal benefit to the millions of Americans already afflicted with the disease. This is a bleak statement, but I think one that is unavoidable. What are its implications?

I wrote in an earlier chapter about what seem to be demographic imperatives we must face as providers of care and as citizens. I alluded to the fact that "Long-term care facilities have always cared for individuals with serious cognitive impairments." What is new is not the fact of the presence of demented old people in our long-term care facilities, but the number and proportion of these individuals.

In the late 1950s, Alvin Goldfarb, in his work for the New York State Department of Mental Hygiene, was one of the first researchers to study empirically and systematically the prevalence of cognitive impairment among the residents of state mental hospitals, not-for-profit homes for the aging, and proprietary nursing homes. Ours was one of the homes which served as a site for Dr. Goldfarb's study, and we, like our colleagues in other facilities he studied, were surprised at the results of his study. Even then, almost three decades ago, we had more impaired older people in our care than we had thought. Residents who tested in the mild to moderate range, whose dementia was not manifested in the kinds of behavior that created management problems, who had devoted families who visited regularly and who were members of strong, interdependent friendship groups within the home, were likely to escape recognition. Often it was only in the later stages, when the impairment could no longer be hidden by dissembling behavior, masked by the resident's social graces, or minimized by loving families, friends, and staff, that the condition was recognized for what it was.

Our staff learned from Dr. Goldfarb about that prevalence of cognitive impairment. We learned about behavioral manifestations of impairment. We also learned about the importance of homes like ours in the service system for the cognitively impaired. Finally, we learned about environmental design and treatment strategies. Now I must share what we and others in long-term care have learned from great pioneers like Dr. Goldfarb and from our own work, because charting the future relies for its foundation on current knowledge and experience.

First is the need for more facilities. Although I recognize that there is disagreement among policy makers, administrators, and researchers on this point, I believe that we must anticipate a future need for more facilities with specialized units or at least a number of beds allocated to demented older people. We ignore demographic trends and indicators of need for more institutional care only at serious risk to America's older population and their families.

Second is the need for less negative bias, which Marion Roach expressed in her introductory chapter: "I did not want to think that my mother would ever end up in a nursing home; I really thought that that's where people got dumped."

Many people in geriatrics and gerontology write about the "institutional bias" built into the Medicaid Title of the Social Security Act. But there is also an "anti-institutional bias" abroad in our land, which Marion's words capture so poignantly. Families struggle nobly to maintain their cognitively impaired member at home, precisely because they share Marion's fear of long-term care facilities as well as her belief that it is here that selfish children abandon their aged parents. Like Marion, they believe that their parents should be spared at all costs the indignity and the stigma of ending up in a nursing home.

The bias, fear, and stigma exist as powerful blocks in the path between the Alzheimer's patient and family and the care and services they need. I do not believe that there will be a sufficient number of facilities providing quality care unless we are able to confront this bias and to help policymakers and families alike truly understand, as Marion has come to, that a home can be a less restrictive environment than an apartment, and that placement can become not the last resort but the arrangement of choice.

Third is the need for staff education. One of the outcomes of Dr. Goldfarb's study was the development of a training program for our staff designed to increase the knowledge and skill of staff from all departments of the home in work with the mentally impaired. It was clear then and is equally clear now that the provision of skilled, humane, intelligent care—care that is the right of all Alzheimer's patients—requires specialized and sophisticated knowledge and skill. Good intentions of staff charged with providing care to our cognitively impaired residents are admirable but not sufficient. Special skills are required to motivate Alzheimer's patients; to help maximize the capabilities that remain; to chart the course of the disease and adjust programs and environments accordingly; to know how to communicate, how to convey concern, how to respond to anger, agitation, and depression; and to do all of the things that form the components of care. These skills must be grounded in knowledge and learned and practiced under careful supervision.

We must invest resources in the continuing and continuous education of our staff. Such an investment will be rewarded in the quality of staff work. In addition, it has at least two other purposes.

If we place hands-on staff in the work situation without proper orientation and without the opportunity for continuing education, then surely we are delivering a message to staff, families, and patients alike: the work of staff is not of sufficient value and the people they care for are not of sufficient human importance to warrant investment in staff training. If anyone can do it, then the care of the demented old person must not be worth doing well. Training promotes not only skill but also professional pride.

Moreover, in our experience training is an effective strategy in reducing staff burnout and the high rates of turnover that plague many facilities. The staff person who receives no guidance in ministering to the needs of a demented and often difficult older person and who senses that there are better ways to do his or her job but is not helped to find those ways is likely to become demoralized and hopeless. Some remain on the job but lose motivation; they go through the motions but without skill or knowledge or eventually even human compassion. Some do not remain; they leave after six months, vowing never to go near sick old people again.

One more thought about the training needs of staff: I came to the field of geriatric care from the children's field, and I have never stopped being amazed at how often cognitively impaired older people are treated like the children I worked with more than 30 years ago. Training that emphasizes the personhood of all residents and includes attention to communication skills—making statements and asking questions, talking in simple sentences, and using the right words—is helpful training. We have found that staff who are poorly trained for the work are those most likely to infantilize and patronize our impaired residents. They are the staff least able to provide the needed care.

Fourth is the need for specialized units. As we chart our direction for the years to come, the necessity for specialized institutions or specialized units within our facilities for those residents who suffer from Alzheimer's and other dementing conditions must be recognized and implemented in our work. The days when separation of physically and cognitively impaired elderly was an arguable point seem to me to be long gone. I recognize the difficulties that small facilities face, but to argue that the intellectually impaired benefit from sharing their living space with the intact and that the intact are well cared for on units designed to protect and sustain the impaired does damage to all. The physical and social environment and the recruitment and training of staff must be specific to the needs of the impaired. An environment that is beneficial for the intellectually able is too rich, too complex, for the impaired. The environment and the staff that Mrs. Roach and others need is stultifying and sterile for those who are physically ill but mentally alert. Let us face this reality and design our facilities in accord with it.

The tasks we face in the future are not easy. The obstacles are real. The bias against institutional care is powerful, yet we have no alternative except to continue and increase our efforts to provide the kind of care those suffering from dementing diseases deserve.

Index

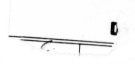